Frontiers in Clinical Neurotoxicology

Guest Editors

MICHAEL R. DOBBS, MD
DANIEL E. RUSYNIAK, MD

NEUROLOGIC CLINICS

www.neurologic.theclinics.com

Consulting Editor
RANDOLPH W. EVANS, MD

August 2011 • Volume 29 • Number 3

SAUNDERS an imprint of ELSEVIER, Inc.

W.B. SAUNDERS COMPANY
A Division of Elsevier Inc.

1600 John F. Kennedy Boulevard • Suite 1800 • Philadelphia, Pennsylvania 19103-2899

http://www.theclinics.com

NEUROLOGIC CLINICS Volume 29, Number 3
August 2011 ISSN 0733-8619, ISBN-13: 978-1-4557-1111-6

Editor: Donald Mumford

Neurologic Clinics (ISSN 0733-8619) is published quarterly by Elsevier Inc., 360 Park Avenue South, New York, NY 10010–1710. Months of issue are February, May, August, and November. Periodicals postage paid at New York, NY, and additional mailing offices. Subscription prices are $264.00 per year for US individuals, $441.00 per year for US institutions, $130.00 per year for US students, $332.00 per year for Canadian individuals, $530.00 per year for Canadian institutions, $368.00 per year for international individuals, $530.00 per year for international institutions, and $184.00 for Canadian and foreign students/residents. To receive student/resident rate, orders must be accompanied by name of affiliated institution, date of term, and the *signature* of program/residency coordinator on institution letterhead. Orders will be billed at individual rate until proof of status is received. Foreign air speed delivery is included in all *Clinics* subscription prices. All prices are subject to change without notice. **POSTMASTER:** Send address changes to *Neurologic Clinics*, Elsevier Health Sciences Division, Subscription Customer Service, 3251 Riverport Lane, Maryland Heights, MO 63043. **Customer Service: Telephone: 1-800-654-2452 (U.S. and Canada); 314-447-8871 (outside U.S. and Canada). Fax: 314-447-8029. E-mail: journalscustomerservice-usa@elsevier.com (for print support); journalsonlinesupport-usa@elsevier.com (for online support).**

Reprints. For copies of 100 or more of articles in this publication, please contact the Commercial Reprints Department, Elsevier Inc., 360 Park Avenue South, New York, New York, 10010-1710; Tel.: (+1) 212-633-3812; Fax: (+1) 212-462-1935, and E-mail: reprints@elsevier.com.

Neurologic Clinics is also published in Spanish by Nueva Editorial Interamericana S.A., Mexico City, Mexico.

Neurologic Clinics is covered in *Current Contents/Clinical Medicine, MEDLINE/PubMed (Index Medicus), EMBASE/Excerpta Medica, and PsycINFO, and ISI/BIOMED.*

Printed and bound by CPI Group (UK) Ltd, Croydon, CR0 4YY

Transferred to Digital Print 2011

Contributors

CONSULTING EDITOR

RANDOLPH W. EVANS, MD
Clinical Professor, Department of Neurology, Baylor College of Medicine, Houston, Texas

GUEST EDITORS

MICHAEL R. DOBBS, MD
Associate Professor and Vice-Chair, Department of Neurology, University of Kentucky College of Medicine, Lexington, Kentucky

DANIEL E. RUSYNIAK, MD
Associate Professor of Emergency Medicine, Adjunct Associate Professor of Pharmacology, Toxicology, and Clinical Neurology, Indiana University School of Medicine, Indianapolis, Indiana

AUTHORS

AIESHA AHMED, MD
Assistant Professor of Neurology, Department of Neurology, Hershey Medical Center, Penn State College of Medicine, Hershey, Pennsylvania

J. DAVE BARRY, MD
Director, Emergency Medicine Residency Program; Department of Emergency Medicine, Naval Medical Center Portsmouth, Portsmouth, Virginia; Assistant Professor of Military and Emergency Medicine, Uniformed Services University of the Health Sciences, Bethesda, Maryland

BRANDON C. DENNIS, PsyD
Neuropsychology Fellow, Department of Neurology, University of Kentucky College of Medicine, Lexington, Kentucky

BRENT FURBEE, MD, FACMT
Medical Director, Indiana Poison Center; Associate Clinical Professor of Emergency Medicine, Division of Medical Toxicology, Department of Emergency Medicine, Indiana University School of Medicine, Indianapolis, Indiana

DONG (DAN) Y. HAN, PsyD
Assistant Professor of Neurology, Department of Neurology, University of Kentucky College of Medicine, Lexington, Kentucky

JAMES B. HOELZLE, PhD
Assistant Professor, Department of Psychology, Marquette University, Milwaukee, Wisconsin

MICHAEL HOFFMANN, MD
Professor of Neurology, Department of Neurology, James A. Haley Veteran's Hospital, Tampa, Florida

ROBERT S. HOFFMAN, MD, FAACT, FACMT, FRCPEdin
Department of Emergency Medicine, New York University School of Medicine, Bellevue Hospital Center, New York, New York

DAVID H. JANG, MD
Department of Emergency Medicine, New York University School of Medicine, Bellevue Hospital Center, New York, New York

DAVID A. JETT, PhD
Program Director, Office of Translational Research, National Institute of Neurological Disorders and Stroke, National Institutes of Health, Bethesda, Maryland

BRYAN S. JUDGE, MD
Associate Program Director, Grand Rapids Medical Education Partners/Michigan State University Emergency Medicine Residency; Associate Professor, Division of Emergency Medicine, Michigan State University College of Human Medicine; Spectrum Health-Toxicology Services, Grand Rapids, Michigan

HANI A. KUSHLAF, MB, BCh
Peripheral Nerve Fellow, Department of Neurology, Mayo Clinic, Rochester, Minnesota

LANDEN L. RENTMEESTER, MD
Assistant Clinical Instructor, Division of Emergency Medicine, Michigan State University College of Human Medicine; Resident Physician, Grand Rapids Medical Education Partners/Michigan State University Emergency Medicine Residency, Grand Rapids, Michigan

DANIEL E. RUSYNIAK, MD
Associate Professor of Emergency Medicine, Adjunct Associate Professor of Pharmacology, Toxicology, and Clinical Neurology, Indiana University School of Medicine, Indianapolis, Indiana

JOHN T. SLEVIN, MD, MBA
Director, Movement Disorders Program; Professor, Departments of Neurology, Molecular and Biomedical Pharmacology, University of Kentucky College of Medicine; Director, Parkinson's Disease Consortium Center, Lexington Veterans Affairs Medical Center, Lexington, Kentucky

LAURA M. TORMOEHLEN, MD
Assistant Professor of Clinical Neurology, Departments of Neurology and Emergency Medicine, Indiana University School of Medicine, Indianapolis, Indiana

MATTHEW P. WICKLUND, MD
Professor of Neurology, Department of Neurology, Hershey Medical Center, Penn State College of Medicine, Hershey, Pennsylvania

BRANDON K. WILLS, DO, MS
Director, Medical Toxicology Fellowship, Virginia Commonwealth University Medical Center; Assistant Professor, Department of Emergency Medicine, Virginia Commonwealth University Health Center; Associated Medical Director, Virginia Poison Center, Richmond, Virginia

FARIHA ZAHEER, MD
Resident in Neurology, Department of Neurology, University of Kentucky College of Medicine, Lexington, Kentucky

Contents

Neurotoxic emergencies are depicted by severe disruption of critical central or peripheral nervous system functions caused by xenobiotics with rapid mechanisms of action. This article reviews 4 categories of neurotoxic emergency: drug-induced and toxin-induced seizures, acute depressed mental status, acute excited mental status, and peripheral neurotoxic agents. Selected xenobiotics, representing the frontiers of neurotoxic emergencies, are discussed in detail based on the major neurotransmitters involved.

Antidepressants are the most commonly prescribed class of medications in the United States. The clinician should be mindful of the many antidepressants that can produce seizures following an accidental exposure or an overdose. A broader understanding of the seizure potential of antidepressants, combined with the ability to recognize individuals at risk for a seizure after an overdose, can aid clinicians in determining the need for inpatient monitoring, and help facilitate their treatment decisions.

Among commercial and industrial chemicals, cosmetics, food additives, pesticides, and medicinal drugs, there are more than 50,000 substances distributed. Neurotoxic insults to the brain can manifest in many different ways, especially involving cognition. Given many possible differences in the pathophysiology of neurotoxic exposure and related cognitive sequelae, a systematic method of cognitive assessment is important for appropriate management of neurotoxic exposure. In the context of Neurotoxicology, this article briefly reviews the contemporary literature and the utility of cognitive assessment tools that are used in neuropsychology.

Leukoencephalopathy is a syndrome of neurologic deficits, including alteration of mental status, caused by pathologic changes in the cerebral white matter. The term, *toxic leukoencephalopathy*, encompasses a wide variety of exposures and clinical presentations. The diagnosis in these

parkinsonian features. Animal and cell culture models indicate mitochondrial dysfunction as the probable mechanism, most likely mediated by TaClo, a potential TCE metabolite. These observations endorse the hypothesis that a variety of environmental risk factors may cause nigrostriatal degeneration and clinical parkinsonism in genetically predisposed individuals.

FORTHCOMING ISSUES

RECENT ISSUES

THE CLINICS ARE NOW AVAILABLE ONLINE!
Access your subscription at:
www.theclinics.com

Preface

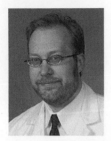 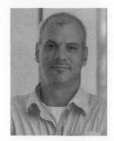

Michael R. Dobbs, MD   Daniel E. Rusyniak, MD
Guest Editors

There are stages in the evolution of medical care for specific conditions as described by Christensen, Grossman, and Hwang in *The Innovator's Prescription—A Disruptive Solution for Health Care.* Typically, a medical disorder emerges in the *intuitive* stage. At this stage only the most skilled, cutting-edge practitioners are able to offer reasonably accurate diagnoses based on a murky amalgam of history, ambiguous exam findings, non-standardized laboratory data, anecdotal case reports in the literature, and elusive personal experience. Treatment in the intuitive medicine arena is typically empiric, utilizing trial and error methods with limited success. Later, as research accumulates and care is standardized, the disorder may move into the *precision* stage. Here, precise diagnosis is possible through standardized, validated tests, and treatments are based on sound clinical trials. Finally, if a disorder is chronic and afflicts a sufficient number of people, the *facilitated networks* stage of disease management becomes possible. Outside of select emergency poisoning syndromes with specific antidotes, most clinical neurotoxicology conditions today fall into the intuitive stage of medicine, and that is what this edition of *Neurologic Clinics* is about.

The questions covered in *Frontiers in Clinical Neurotoxicology* are really out there on the edge. In some cases, there are so few practitioners well-versed in these disorders that it was nearly impossible to find authors. However, you will find as you read the articles that we found excellent and experienced practitioners and scientists to contribute. You will learn valuable lessons by reading their work, and we hope that you can carry some of these lessons to your clinical practice. Our authors hail from medical toxicology, neurology, emergency medicine, and cognitive and other basic sciences. Some contributors are still in training and could represent the future of clinical neurotoxicology practice.

We would like to thank the contributors to this issue as well as our friends at Elsevier. Don Mumford at Elsevier was patient and helpful with putting this issue together. We also want to thank the readers for carrying the torch and helping us to move toward *precision* in clinical neurotoxicology. Together we will strive to develop reliable

Neurol Clin 29 (2011) xi–xii
doi:10.1016/j.ncl.2011.06.003
0733-8619/11/$ – see front matter © 2011 Elsevier Inc. All rights reserved.

diagnostic and treatment routines for the millions of people who suffer from neurotoxic problems.

Michael R. Dobbs, MD
Department of Neurology
University of Kentucky College of Medicine
740 South Limestone Street
Wing D, KY Clinic
Lexington, KY 40536, USA

Daniel E. Rusyniak, MD
Department of Emergency Medicine
Indiana University School of Medicine
1050 Wishard Boulevard, Room 2200
Indianapolis, IN 46202, USA

E-mail addresses:
mrdobb0@email.uky.edu (M.R. Dobbs)
drusynia@iupui.edu (D.E. Rusyniak)

Neurotoxic Emergencies

J. Dave Barry, MD[a,b,c,]*, Brandon K. Wills, DO, MS[d,e,f]

KEYWORDS

• Poisoning • Emergency • Overdose • Neurology • Toxicology

The symptoms and effects delineating a neurotoxic emergency vary depending on the viewpoint of the clinician. In general, agents causing acute life-threatening conditions have rapid mechanisms that severely disrupt major organ systems. This article focuses on agents causing rapid decompensation to a potentially life-threatening condition. The majority of these agents affect the central nervous system (CNS), thus the article is structured based on CNS effects: drug-induced and toxin-induced seizures, acute depressed mental status, and acute excited mental status. The final section highlights selected agents with primarily peripheral effects that meet the same criteria for an acute life-threatening condition.

A wide variety of poisons, toxins, drugs, chemicals, industrial agents, pesticides, and environmental agents have the potential to cause emergent neurotoxic effects. To avoid confusion, the authors use the term "xenobiotic" when discussing the various causative neurotoxic agents. A xenobiotic is a pharmacologically, endocrinologically, or toxicologically active substance not endogenously produced and therefore foreign to the organism.[1]

Neurotoxic xenobiotics produce symptoms in the victim through a wide array of different mechanisms, as shown in **Table 1**. Neurotoxic emergencies frequently affect the CNS through effects on neurotransmitters; therefore, much of this discussion focuses on the actions of specific neurotransmitters.

The views expressed in this article are those of the authors and do not reflect the official policy, position, or doctrine of the US Army, US Navy, DOD, or the US Government.

The authors have nothing to disclose.

[a] Emergency Medicine Residency Program, Naval Medical Center Portsmouth, Portsmouth, VA, USA

[b] Department of Emergency Medicine, Naval Medical Center Portsmouth, 620 John Paul Jones Circle, Portsmouth, VA 23708-2197, USA

[c] Uniformed Services University of the Health Sciences, Bethesda, MD, USA

[d] Virginia Commonwealth University Medical Center, Richmond, VA, USA

[e] Department of Emergency Medicine, Virginia Commonwealth University Health Center, Richmond, VA, USA

[f] Virginia Poison Center, PO Box 980522, Richmond, VA 23298, USA

* Corresponding author. 2605 Admiral Drive, Virginia Beach, VA 23451.

E-mail address: James.barry@med.navy.mil

Neurol Clin 29 (2011) 539–563

doi:10.1016/j.ncl.2011.05.006

0733-8619/11/$ – see front matter. Published by Elsevier Inc.

neurologic.theclinics.com

Table 1	
Mechanisms of neurotoxic xenobiotics	
Effect	**Specific Mechanism**
Cellular	Oxidative stress (free radicals, nucleophiles, or electrophiles)
	Alteration of membrane integrity
	Disruption of energy metabolism and/or regulation
	Altered regulation of gene expression
	Altered protein production
	Disruption of intracellular ion homeostasis
Metabolic	Stimulation or inhibition of enzymatic function
	Mimicking the actions of nutrients, hormones, or neurotransmitters
Neurotransmitter	Stimulation or blockade neurotransmitter receptors
	Altered release, uptake, and/or storage of neurotransmitters
	Altered neurotransmitter production or metabolism

DRUG-INDUCED AND TOXIN-INDUCED SEIZURES

Seizures are a manifestation of many drug and toxin exposures or withdrawal syndromes. Some overdoses may include seizure amongst a myriad of other organ system toxicities, whereas others induce seizures as the primary manifestation of toxicity. Drug-induced and toxin-induced seizures (DTS) are typically generalized seizures, with status epilepticus occurring in approximately 4% to 10% of cases.[2,3] The epidemiology and incidence of DTS are not well known because seizures are not always tracked by regional poison centers. The California Poison Control Systems have provided the best view of agents most frequently implicated in DTS through a series of investigations over the last 17 years.[2–4] Over this time period, the proportion of DTS from tricyclic antidepressants (TCA), stimulants, and theophylline fell while anticholinergic antihistamines and isoniazid remained fairly constant. Their most recent prospective series of DTS found antidepressants were most common (33%) followed by stimulants (15%), antiepileptics (12%), and anticholinergic antihistamines (10%).[2] Of note, citalopram and escitalopram were absent from their 1994 and 2003 series yet comprised 8% of cases in the most recent review.[2] A comprehensive review of toxin-related seizures was recently published.[5] This section discusses some of the more common and newer pharmaceuticals implicated in DTS.

Psychiatric Agents

Tricyclic antidepressants

TCAs have multiple pharmacologic effects including serotonin and norepinephrine reuptake inhibition, central and peripheral anticholinergic and antihistamine effects, peripheral α_1 antagonism, and fast sodium channel blockade.[6] A recent series documenting prevalence of clinical outcomes in amitriptyline overdose reported seizures in 6%, hypotension in 10%, coma in 29%, and wide QRS complex or ventricular dysrhythmia in 30%.[7] Acidemia from seizures or hypotension can decrease TCA protein binding, resulting in worsening toxicity.[8] Seizures are treated primarily with benzodiazepines. Boluses of sodium bicarbonate are useful for the cardiovascular effects of TCA poisoning by providing a sodium bolus as well as raising the serum pH.[6,8]

Bupropion

Bupropion is a mixed dopamine and norepinephrine reuptake inhibitor, well known to lower the seizure threshold in therapeutic doses and induce seizures in overdose.[9] Of all drug-induced seizures reported to a regional poison center, 14.9% were due to bupropion.[2] Another poison center review of bupropion overdoses reported generalized seizures in 32% of cases, 32% of which occurred more than 8 hours after overdose.[10] In this series, 19% of patients who seized also exhibited hallucinations. One patient did not manifest their first seizure until 24 hours after ingestion.

Citalopram

Citalopram overdose is frequently associated with QTc prolongation and seizures.[11] One 7-year review found seizures in 8% of citalopram overdoses; however, nearly half of the cases involved coingestants.[12] Escitalopram is the S-enantiomer of citalopram and produces substantially fewer seizures in overdose.[13,14]

Antiepileptic drugs

Seizures can paradoxically occur from overdose of anticonvulsants. This phenomenon is unlikely to occur in γ-aminobutyric acid (GABA)-mediated anticonvulsants but is seen in anticonvulsants with mixed receptor effects. Traditional anticonvulsants known to cause seizures in overdose are carbamazepine and, to a lesser extent, phenytoin.[15–17] The authors have less clinical experience with newer anticonvulsants, but seizures appear to occur frequently in overdose. Lamotrigine has been associated with seizures and nonconvulsive status epilepticus in both therapeutic dosing[18–20] and overdose.[21,22] Topirimate[23,24] and tiagabine[25–27] have also been reported to cause seizures in overdose.

Drugs of Abuse

Acute intoxication or drug withdrawal from several different classes can result in seizures. The stimulant class includes a diverse range of illicit drugs including amphetamines (illicit and medicinal), designer amphetamines, cocaine, and methylxanthines. Manifestations of stimulant overdose include a sympathomimetic toxidrome manifested by tachycardia, hypertension, mydriasis, diaphoresis, agitation, and tremor. Generalized seizures are frequently seen in moderate to severe cases.[28–30] Methylxanthine overdose can manifest with significant tachycardia, hypotension rather than hypertension, dysrhythmias, and refractory seizures.[29] Animal models and human series suggest hyperthermia in the setting of stimulant overdose is a surrogate of severe poisoning and increased mortality.[31–34]

The sympathomimetic toxidrome is frequently seen in moderate to severe sedative-hypnotic withdrawal. Seizures from drug withdrawal are observed primarily with ethanol,[35] sedative-hypnotics (eg, benzodiazepines, barbiturates), and baclofen.[36–38] It is uncommon for opioid withdrawal to cause seizures except in neonates born to opioid-dependent mothers.[39]

Opioids

The vast majority of opioids do not cause seizures in acute overdose or in withdrawal. A few notable exceptions are discussed here.

Tramadol

Tramadol is a synthetic analgesic with weak μ-receptor effects as well as serotonin and norepinephrine reuptake inhibition.[40] Case series of tramadol overdoses documented generalized seizures in 8% to 54% of cases, 45% to 63% being single seizures.[41–43] Other complications include rhabdomyolysis, acute kidney injury, and serotonin toxicity.[44,45]

Propoxyphene

Overdose of propoxyphene in some ways can mimic tricyclic antidepressant overdose with CNS depression, wide-complex dysrhythmias due to fast sodium channel blockade, and seizures.[46–48] In November 2010, propoxyphene was removed from United States markets, and removal has been under way since 2009 across Europe.

Meperidine
Meperidine, a synthetic opioid, is demethylated to the neurotoxic metabolite normeperidine.[49] Patients with renal insufficiency or receiving continuous infusions through patient-controlled analgesia devices are at particular risk for neurotoxicity and seizures.[50]

Other Agents

Isoniazid
Isoniazid (INH), a hydrazine used for tuberculosis, is well known for causing refractory seizures in overdose. Hydrazines can also be found in some types of rocket fuel and in the toxic mushroom *Gyromitra esculenta*. Hydrazines inhibit pyridoxine phosphokinase resulting in a functional vitamin B6 deficiency, an essential cofactor for GABA synthesis. INH overdose may include the triad of coma, severe lactic acidosis, and refractory seizures.[51]

Treatment

Decontamination considerations
Gastrointestinal decontamination options include gastric lavage, activated charcoal, and whole bowel irrigation. Gastric lavage is generally not recommended for most overdoses.[52] Single-dose activated charcoal is theoretically effective for most organic substances except for metals, hydrocarbons, alcohols, and caustics. Its efficacy for preventing absorption drops off sharply by 2 to 3 hours post ingestion.[53] Activated charcoal is contraindicated for patients with CNS depression, significant delirium, high risk for seizures, or an unprotected airway due to risks of pulmonary aspiration.[53] Whole bowel irrigation (WBI) involves the administration of polyethylene glycol solution at a rate of 1 to 2 liters per hour until the rectal effluent is clear. Although WBI has theoretical advantages for substances not absorbed by activated charcoal and sustained-release products, its routine use is not currently recommended.[54] It is also difficult to achieve complete bowel decontamination.[55] As mentioned with activated charcoal, neurotoxic overdoses resulting in alteration of consciousness and seizures increase the risk of pulmonary aspiration.

Enhanced elimination considerations
Enhancing the elimination of drugs or toxins can be accomplished through multidose activated charcoal (MDAC), urinary alkalinization, and hemodialysis. Drug overdoses likely to cause seizures that are amenable to MDAC include theophylline, carbamazepine, and quinine.[56] As with single-dose activated charcoal, patients with seizures or unprotected airway represent a significant risk for aspiration. Urinary alkalinization involves the administration of bicarbonate to raise urine pH above 7.5. It is useful to enhance the elimination of salicylates in moderate to severe poisonings.[57] Hemodialysis is also useful for moderate to severe toxicity from salicylates, lithium, and theophylline overdoses.[58]

Focused treatment
Initial management of the seizing patient includes attention to the airway, breathing, and circulation; establishing peripheral intravenous access, starting supplemental oxygen, bedside glucose determination, giving empiric anticonvulsant therapy, and treating other underlying sequelae due to overdose (eg, rhabdomyolysis or

hyperthermia). Consultation with a medical toxicologist is useful for providing guidance on decontamination, enhanced elimination, resuscitative interventions, and antidotes.

DTS, which are frequently short lived and self limited, may not require anticonvulsant therapy. However, approximately 4% to 10% of DTS result in status epilepticus.[2,3] Evidence-based approaches to treating drugs and DTS are lacking. Recommendations are frequently extrapolated from epilepsy research, pharmacologic mechanisms, and anecdotal experience. For most cases of DTS, anticonvulsant treatment should be focused on GABA agonists. Benzodiazepines remain first-line therapy for DTS. Lorazepam or diazepam are generally preferred, but barbiturates can also be used. Unlike seizures from drug overdose, severe delirium tremens may require massive doses of benzodiazepines to achieve control.[59,60] Propofol is an intravenous anesthetic that has been effective in controlling severe delirium tremens refractory to other agents.[61,62] It may be tried as a second-line therapy for refractory DTS.[63,64]

Phenytoin should not be considered first-line or second-line therapy for DTS. Phenytoin is not expected to be effective for the majority of DTS, and may exacerbate seizures with cocaine, lidocaine, theophylline, and organochlorine insecticides.[65] There is little evidence regarding the efficacy of valproic acid or levetiracetam for DTS, but because they have been used for non-DTS status epilepticus, are well tolerated, available as an intravenous bolus, and are GABA agonists, they would be reasonable to try as a third-line therapy.[66] One murine model evaluated 13 anticonvulsants' ability to prevent seizures induced by bupropion.[67] The investigators determined that carbamazepine, lamotrigine, phenytoin, and tiagabine were not effective at attenuating seizures.

Pyridoxine is indicated for isoniazid overdose with either seizure or coma.[68] It is given as an empiric dose of 5 g or at a dose equivalent to the amount of INH ingested if this is known.[69]

ACUTE DEPRESSED MENTAL STATUS

Chemical balance within the CNS is principally maintained by GABA as the predominant inhibitory neurotransmitter and by glutamate, the predominant excitatory neurotransmitter.[70] A wide variety of other neurotransmitters, ion channels, and modulators contribute in a less significant way to this balance, and are less understood. Stimulation by GABA, γ-hydroxybutyrate (GHB), opioids, and cannabinoids all have the potential to produce acute depressed mental status.

γ-Aminobutyric Acid

There are 3 distinct GABA receptor subtypes: $GABA_A$, $GABA_B$, and $GABA_C$. $GABA_A$ receptors are ligand-gated chloride ion channels. In addition to the GABA binding sites, there are others where multiple xenobiotics and endogenous modulators can bind, altering the chloride current. Xenobiotics causing acute depressed mental status commonly target this $GABA_A$ receptor complex. $GABA_B$ are G-protein–coupled receptors that ultimately alter calcium or potassium currents.[71] $GABA_C$ are ligand-gated chloride ion channels that are structurally, functionally, and pharmacologically distinct from $GABA_A$.[72] The clinical importance of $GABA_C$ receptors is poorly understood.

Neurotoxic xenobiotics can alter GABA homeostasis, leading to acute depressed mental status in a variety of ways. The most common mechanism is through indirect stimulation of $GABA_A$ receptors, increasing the affinity of GABA for its receptor, or increasing the frequency or duration of chloride channel opening. Both benzodiazepine and barbiturate classes of drugs,[73–76] steroids,[76] various anesthetics,[76] and other xenobiotics exert their clinical effects through these mechanisms. Muscimol, a direct

GABA$_A$ agonist, is found naturally in *Aminita muscaria* (fly agaric) and *Aminita pantherina* (panther cap) mushrooms, along with ibotenic acid, an excitatory glutamic acid receptor agonist.[77] Baclofen is a direct GABA$_B$ receptor agonist. Commonly administered via an intrathecal pump, baclofen overdose can cause profound CNS depression.[78]

GABA concentrations in the brain can be increased by stimulating GABA production, regulated by the enzyme glutamic acid decarboxylase (GAD) or by decreasing GABA metabolism, regulated by GABA transaminase. These mechanisms contribute at least partially to the clinical effects of sodium valproate,[79,80] gabapentin,[81] and vigabatrin.[82] Tiagabine similarly increases GABA concentrations by inhibiting GABA reuptake through blockade of the GABA transporter, GAT-1.[83]

Treatment of acute depressed mental status caused by GABA stimulation is primarily supportive, with specific attention to the patient's protective airway reflexes, and ventilatory and oxygenation status. Flumazenil binds to the benzodiazepine site on the GABA receptor, competitively inhibiting benzodiazepines and related xenobiotics. Although flumazenil effectively reverses the CNS effects of these agents,[84] it is not recommended for routine use on all altered or comatose patients because of the potential for inducing withdrawal in the chronic user, provoking seizures in both epileptic and nonepileptic patients, and unmasking excitatory coingestants. Reasonable use of flumazenil would be in benzodiazepine overdose in naïve patients and iatrogenic benzodiazepine overdose from procedural sedation.[85]

γ-Hydroxybutyrate

GHB is an endogenous neurotransmitter. Marketed as sodium oxybate, a pharmaceutical treatment for narcolepsy, it is also a popular drug of abuse. GHB is both a precursor and a metabolite of GABA. Structurally similar, these compounds share a common catabolic and metabolic pathway. GHB precursors are widely used in industry, but are also commonly abused recreationally as food supplements, and are rarely implicated as incapacitating agents (facilitating sexual assault).[86]

Although similar to GABA, GHB has its own distinct G-protein–linked receptor. The mechanisms of action of GHB are incompletely understood. Whether through interactions at the GHB receptor or by neuromodulation at other receptors, GHB alters CNS concentrations of GABA, dopamine, serotonin, norepinephrine, opioids, and glutamate.[87,88]

Physiologic concentrations of GHB interact primarily at the GHB receptors.[88] The administration of exogenous GHB, either for therapeutic or recreational reasons, dramatically increases CNS concentrations. The effects of supraphysiologic GHB concentrations are primarily mediated at GABA$_B$ receptors, but additional less well described interactions probably also occur.[87–89]

Supraphysiologic GHB concentrations produce varying degrees of CNS depression ranging from disinhibition (agitated delirium), to mild (sedation, ataxia, dizziness), to severe (coma, respiratory depression, apnea, death).[90–92] Other common symptoms include bradycardia, hypothermia, and vomiting. Myoclonus and convulsive activity has been reported with GHB toxicity, but it is unclear whether these are true seizures.[90,93] Abrupt awakening from deep coma is commonly reported in association with GHB toxicity.[94] With chronic use, a withdrawal syndrome, clinically similar to sedative-hypnotic withdrawal, can manifest after abrupt discontinuation.

Treatment of GHB toxicity is primarily symptomatic and supportive. Various agents (flumazenil, naloxone, physostigmine) have been suggested as antidotes for GHB toxicity, but none have shown consistent efficacy. GHB withdrawal is treated in a similar fashion to sedative-hypnotic withdrawal, with high-dose benzodiazepine as the first-line agent. Refractory GHB withdrawal has been described. These cases can be controlled with cross-tolerant sedative-hypnotics such as benzodiazepines, barbiturates, chloral hydrate, or propofol.[95,96] Baclofen has also been suggested as a treatment for GHB withdrawal.[97]

Opioids

Opioid receptors are distributed widely throughout the CNS, spinal cord, and peripheral nervous system (PNS). Although extensively studied, the clinical effects mediated by their G-protein–mediated receptors are not completely understood. The classic Greek nomenclature (μ, κ, δ) used to describe opioid receptors is transitioning to one recommended by the International Union on Receptor Nomenclature (MOP/ OP_3, KOP/OP_2, DOP/OP_1). There are 3 primary opioid receptors, each with their own specific subtypes, and a few less well described minor receptors. Each receptor type is distributed differently throughout the human body and imparts different clinical effects.

The μ (mu) opioid receptor (MOP, OP_3) was the first to be described as the morphine-binding site and is probably the best understood. Although there are 2 distinct subtypes (μ_1/OP_{3A}, μ_2/OP_{3B}), there are no known selective subtype xenobiotics. μ receptors mediate most of the clinical effects commonly attributed to opioids: analgesia, euphoria, sedation, respiratory depression, decreased gastrointestinal motility, and physical dependence.[98] κ (kappa) opioid receptors (KOP, OP_2) are concentrated in the spinal cord, mediating primarily spinal analgesia, miosis, and dysphoria. δ (delta) receptors (DOP, OP_1) are less well understood but may contribute to the psychomimetic and dysphoric properties of opioids. A fourth nonclassic opioid receptor, the nociceptin/orphanin FQ receptor (NOP, OP_4), was defined using DNA sequencing, but a clinical role has not yet been described.[98,99]

Pure opioid agonists frequently produce acute depressed mental status in conjunction with the classic opioid toxic syndrome: CNS depression, respiratory depression, and miosis.[100] Some opioid xenobiotics possess additional mechanisms of action (meperidine, tramadol, propoxyphene, dextromethorphan), thus the toxic presentation may include symptoms not classic for opioids and/or lack some symptoms of the classic opioid toxidrome.

Treatment of opioid toxicity focuses on early support of ventilation and oxygenation in addition to symptomatic care. Gastrointestinal decontamination should be considered based on the clinical situation. Opioid antagonists competitively inhibit the binding of opioid agonists to opioid receptors. Having a higher affinity for opioid receptors than opioid xenobiotics, they reverse the clinical effects of most opioid agonists.[98,101] Naloxone is the most commonly used opioid antagonist. The goal of opioid antagonist therapy is to restore adequate spontaneous ventilation and ensure that protective airway reflexes remain intact, while avoiding precipitation of acute withdrawal. Thus, the lowest possible dose that allows for adequate oxygenation and airway protection should be used.

Cannabinoids

Tetrahydrocannabinol (Δ^9-THC), cannabidiol (CBD), and cannabinol (CBN) are the most prevalent natural cannabinoids or phytocannabinoids, with the most potent being Δ^9-THC. Although categorized as a CNS depressant, it is extremely uncommon for cannabinoid toxicity to cause acute depressed mental status significant enough to be considered a neurotoxic emergency. Over the last few years, however, there has been resurgence in interest in cannabinoids due to the popularity of synthetic cannabinoid use.

Synthetic cannabinoids have become a popular "legal high," usually in the form of herbal blends purportedly sprayed with potent synthetic cannabinoids. Initially the most common herbal blends were sold under the brand name "spice." Recently, this term seems to have become short-hand for a variety of similar products containing synthetic cannabinoids (Genie, K2, Spice Diamond, Spice Gold, Spice Silver, Yucatan Fire, Zohai, and so forth).[102] These products are marketed as incense blends, avoiding regulatory drug control.[102,103] Synthetic cannabinoids are reported to be more potent than their phytocannabinoid cousins.[102] Attributing the symptoms and complications of "spice" use to synthetic cannabinoids is difficult, due to the different combinations of additives used in these products.

Two distinct cannabinoid receptors have been characterized (CB1, CB2), both of which are G-protein–mediated receptors (GPMR). Globally, CB1 receptors are localized primarily in the brain, spinal cord, and testis, where the CB2 receptors are localized peripherally in immune tissues: leukocytes, splenocytes, and microglia.[104–106] Within the CNS, the cannabinoid system is thought to act as a negative feedback mechanism to dampen synaptic release of both excitatory and inhibitory neurotransmitters including glutamate, GABA, noradrenaline, dopamine, serotonin (5-HT), acetylcholine, and opioids.[106–108] Cannabinoid receptors are the most prevalent GPMR in the brain, with the highest concentrations in the basal ganglia and cerebellum.[106,108]

Cannabinoids have a linear dose-response relationship for inducing neuropsychiatric effects,[107,109,110] which can result in a higher propensity for adverse effects using potent synthetic cannabinoids. At moderate doses, cannabinoids cause CNS depressant effects, including analgesia, euphoria, sedation, anxiolysis, and impairment of cognitive and psychomotor performance.[107–109] Although clinically significant acute toxicity is uncommon, large doses of cannabinoids can lead to adverse psychological effects primarily manifested by anxiety, panic attacks, agitation, acute psychosis, and paranoia.[107,109,111] Peripheral effects include dry mouth, palpitations, tachycardia, and postural hypotension.[109]

Tolerance to the effects of cannabinoids is fairly well described.[107,108] Although psychiatric illness is associated with chronic cannabis use, there is no evidence that this relationship is causal.[106,108] A mild withdrawal syndrome has been demonstrated after cessation of heavy cannabinoid use manifested by the following: cravings, anorexia, insomnia, weight loss, irritability, restlessness, and autonomic effects.[107,108,110,112]

ACUTE EXCITED MENTAL STATUS

Although glutamic acid is the predominant excitatory neurotransmitter in the CNS, its interactions with xenobiotics are less well understood than those of the central biogenic amines. Multiple xenobiotics producing acute excited mental status interact with the central biogenic amines, leading to a variety of toxic syndromes discussed here. The complex and incompletely understood interactions of glutamic acid are then addressed.

Central Biogenic Amines

There are 5 biogenic amine neurotransmitters: histamine, 5-HT, and the 3 catecholamines dopamine (DA), norepinephrine (NE), and epinephrine (EPI). All 5 share common and incompletely understood interactions within the CNS. EPI and histamine have less predominant interactions, ultimately mediating CNS-excited mental status, so they are not discussed in this section.

NE, DA, and 5-HT share similar synthesis, storage, and degradation pathways within the CNS. DA is produced from tyrosine intracellularly in a 2-step enzymatic process involving tyrosine hydroxylase and amino acid decarboxylase. 5-HT utilizes a parallel process, with tryptamine instead of tyrosine as the parent compound. DA β-hydroxylase converts DA to NE after packaging into the nerve-ending vesicles. All 3 are removed from the synapse into the nerve ending by specific reuptake transporters. Although these transporters have high affinity for their parent compounds, they are also somewhat nonspecific, facilitating the transport of similarly structured amines and xenobiotics as well. After reuptake into the synapse, degradation of NE, DA, and 5-HT is primarily performed by monoamine oxidase (MAO).

Receptors for NE, DA, and 5-HT are widely distributed throughout the body. At least 9 different subtypes of NE receptor have been identified,[113] but only α_2 adrenergic receptors play a dominant central role. There are 5 distinct but closely related G-protein–coupled DA receptors, all with broad expression patterns peripherally and centrally.[114] Similarly, 5-HT has 7 major classes of receptor and multiple subtypes.[71] With the exception of 5-HT$_3$ receptors, which are ligand-gated ion channels, all 5-HT receptors are coupled to G proteins.[115]

Amphetamines

Amphetamines and the diverse group of phenethylamine analogues exert their effects indirectly by stimulating NE, DA, and/or 5-HT release, by blocking the reuptake of neurotransmitter into the neuron, and by inhibiting MAO.[116,117] Modifications of the amphetamine structure influence which neurotransmitter is predominantly affected. Amphetamine analogues with prominent serotonergic activity, such as 3,4-methylenedioxymethamphetamine (MDMA, "ecstasy"), yield more intense hallucinogenic properties. Mescaline, the active alkaloid in peyote (*Lophophora williamsii*), shares similar serotonergic effects.[118]

Recently, the synthetic amphetamine analogues mephedrone and methylenedioxypyrovalerone (MDPV) have been found in products sold as "novelty bath salts" ("ivory wave", "vanilla sky", and so forth) on Web sites and in specialty stores.[119] These products share structural similarity with cathinone, the active ingredient in the *Catha edulis* plant (Khat). Metcathinone ("cat", "jeff") is also a synthetic analogue of cathinone.[120]

Cocaine

Similar to amphetamines, cocaine exerts its effects by blocking the reuptake of biogenic amines and thus increasing levels in the nerve terminal.[100,121] Cocaine also increases the concentration of excitatory amino acids,[122] possibly contributing to its clinical effects. Unlike amphetamines, cocaine also possess sodium channel blocking effects (Class I antiarrhythmic) similar to cyclic antidepressants, increasing the risk for cardiac dysrhythmias.[30,121]

Indolealkylamines

Indolealkylamines, or tryptamines, share structural similarity with 5-HT, making this class potent hallucinogens. Psilocybin-containing mushrooms ("magic mushrooms"), 5-methoxy-*N*,*N*-diisopropyltryptamine ("Foxy", "Foxy methoxy"), *N*,*N*-dimethyltryptamine (DMT, Ayahuasca, "Businessman's Lunch"), and α-methyltryptamine (AMT, "spirals") all share similar properties due to their common tryptamine-like structure. Lysergic acid diethylamide (LSD) and its analogues, like those found in morning glory seeds (*Ipomea violacea*), also share structural similarities to 5-HT.[100]

Treatment considerations

Treatment of acute excited mental status due to biogenic amines is symptom and side-effect directed. Hyperthermia should be aggressively treated with active cooling and aggressive control of agitation. Benzodiazepines are first-line agents for agitation and signs of peripheral sympathetic stimulation (tachycardia, hypertension, tachypnea). Alternative GABA agonists (short-acting barbiturates, propofol) can be used for intractable agitation. Persistent hypertension should be controlled with phentolamine or nitrates (nitroglycerine, nitroprusside). Although controversial, β-adrenergic blockers are relatively contraindicated as the resultant unopposed α-adrenergic effects may worsen coronary vasospasm and end-organ toxicity.[123–125] Wide-complex tachydysrhythmias should be treated with sodium bicarbonate. Gastrointestinal decontamination with activated charcoal could be considered for early ingestions. Contraindications are similar to those discussed for seizures. Finally, diligence in watching for and preventing other complications, including rhabdomyolysis, subarachnoid or intraparenchymal hemorrhage, myocardial ischemia, ischemic bowel, and other end-organ effects, is warranted.

Neuroleptic Malignant Syndrome

Neuroleptic malignant syndrome (NMS) is a relatively rare, but potentially fatal complication of treatment with antipsychotic drugs characterized by altered mental status (AMS) (ranging from lethargy, agitation, stupor, to coma), muscle rigidity (classically described as "lead pipe" rigidity[126–128]), fever, and autonomic dysfunction (including tachycardia, tachypnea, hypertension or hypotension, diaphoresis, and possibly cardiac arrhythmias). NMS is usually associated with rapid escalation of an antipsychotic or sudden discontinuation of antiparkinson medications. Neuromuscular manifestations are due to decreased dopaminergic neurotransmission or DA_2 blockade in various CNS locations.[128–130] Symptoms develop over a period of 1 to 3 days, usually in a sequential fashion, beginning with AMS and muscle rigidity.[130]

Initial treatment focuses on early recognition and prompt withdrawal of any dopamine antagonists along with aggressive supportive care, benzodiazepines, and active cooling measures. Dopamine agonists (bromocriptine or amantadine) and dantrolene sodium (based on its efficacy in malignant hyperthermia) have been used anecdotally with varying benefits, but neither has been shown to be consistently superior to supportive care alone.[129–131] Nondepolarizing neuromuscular blockade and mechanical ventilation may be necessary to control rigidity and hyperthermia in severe cases. Electroconvulsive therapy has been performed in patients exhibiting resistant symptoms with anecdotal improvement.[127,129,130] NMS should be considered a diagnosis of exclusion and requires a thorough investigation for alternative causes of AMS, fever, and/or muscle rigidity.

Serotonin Toxicity

Serotonin toxicity is a similar syndrome, characterized by AMS (confusion, agitation, anxiety, hallucinations, lethargy, coma), autonomic instability (flushing, shivering, hypertension, hyperthermia, tachycardia, tachypnea), and neuromuscular abnormalities (tremor, hyperreflexia, myoclonus, muscular rigidity).[132] The manifestations of serotonin toxicity can vary across a spectrum of severity, with the most extreme resembling NMS. Hyperreflexia and clonus in serotonin toxicity are characteristic, being noticeably greater in the lower extremities than in the upper extremities.[126] Unlike NMS, the symptoms occur rapidly, within hours after the initiation of a serotonergic agent, and can escalate quickly to a life-threatening condition.[126,133] The syndrome is thought to be due to increases in extracellular concentrations of serotonin with subsequent stimulation of $5-HT_{2A}$ and other serotonin and monoaminergic receptors.[126,132–134] Although several diagnostic criteria have been proposed,[133,135] these investigators recommend against using them in clinical practice because it could cause oversight and thus delay treatment of atypical cases. Instead, a low threshold should be maintained for diagnosing serotonin toxicity in any patient taking serotonergic xenobiotics that develops a combination of AMS, autonomic findings, and neuromuscular abnormality. Treatment intensity can be tailored to symptom severity but should include discontinuation any serotonergic agents and supportive care. Supportive measures include benzodiazepines for autonomic overactivity and active cooling for hyperthermia. Vasoactive medications, nondepolarizing neuromuscular blockade, and mechanical ventilation may be necessary in severe cases. 5-HT$_{2A}$ antagonists (cyproheptadine, chlorpromazine) have been suggested as adjuncts in moderate to severe cases, but their benefit in humans is largely anectdotal.[126,133]

Glutamic Acid

As mentioned previously, glutamic acid is the predominant excitatory neurotransmitter in the CNS. Glutamic acid is the immediate precursor to GABA, the predominant inhibitory CNS neurotransmitter. Glutamate is closely regulated by the brain, which dedicates up to two-thirds of its energy metabolism to control the reuptake and recycling of this neurotransmitter.[136] There are 11 different types of glutamate receptor: 8 are G-protein mediated (metabotropic), the other 3 being ligand-gated ion channels (ionotropic). The ionotropic receptors are named after the agonist used to identify them. Of these, the N-methyl-D-aspartic acid (NMDA) receptor is the most thoroughly studied. A unique aspect of the NMDA receptor is that it is gated both by ligands and by voltage.[137,138] Magnesium binds to a site within the ion channel, blocking the flow of calcium across the neuronal membrane.[136] In addition to glutamate binding sites, the NMDA channel also has sites for the inhibitory neurotransmitter glycine.[137] The glycine site, similar to the indirect stimulation of GABA receptors, alters the affinity of NMDA for glutamate and varies the frequency or duration of channel opening, but does not, by itself, induce channel opening.[136]

Phencyclidine, Ketamine, Dextromethorphan

Phencyclidine (PCP), ketamine, and dextromethorphan (DXM) bind to an independent site (the PCP binding site)[139] on the NMDA receptor, inhibiting ionic flow. The clinical effects of this inhibition is a "dissociative effect," causing a dissociation between the thalamoneocortical and limbic systems, and preventing the higher centers from perceiving visual, auditory, or painful stimuli.[140] Muscle tone is maintained; therefore, airway protective measures are preserved. In addition to profound anesthetic and analgesic effects, mild cardiovascular stimulation (tachycardia, hypertension, diaphoresis),[140,141] and horizontal, vertical, or rotatory nystagmus[142] are frequently seen. Anxiety, agitation, combativeness, coma, neuromuscular rigidity, and seizures are associated with high doses and/or coingestion of other neuroactive xenobiotics. Hallucinations and nightmares can be seen as subjects emerge from their dissociation; an effect coined as the "emergence phenomenon."[140,142] Treatment is essentially supportive, with benzodiazepine sedation if necessary. The development or coexistence of complications, such as rhabdomyolysis, hyperthermia, acute traumatic injuries, and other end-organ damage, should be pursued. Activated charcoal could benefit patients early after ingestion. In the case of PCP, activated charcoal may also decrease gastroenteric recirculation, shortening the effective half-life.[142]

Domoic Acid

Domoic acid is a neurotoxin, structurally similar to glutamic acid, responsible for amnestic shellfish poisoning (ASP). Domoic acid is produced naturally by various strains of phytoplankton, and is subsequently bioconcentrated by shellfish and finfish (cockles, crabs, furrow shell, mussels, razor clams, scallops) before being inadvertently ingested by humans.[143,144] Domoic acid appears to act as a glutamic acid agonist at all 3 ionotropic glutamate receptors (NMDA, 2-amino-3-(5-methyl-3-oxo-1, 2-oxazol-4-yl)propanoic acid [AMPA], kainate).[144] Ingestion produces gastrointestinal symptoms (nausea, vomiting, abdominal cramps, diarrhea) and neurologic complaints (headache, short-term memory loss). Severe poisoning leads to profound neurologic disturbances including hemiparesis, seizures, coma, and autonomic instability.[143] Treatment is supportive.

PERIPHERAL NEUROTOXIC AGENTS

Although both acetylcholine and glycine are well represented in the CNS, many of their xenobiotic interactions produce effects predominantly expressed in the PNS. In this section, the authors discuss xenobiotics producing PNS effects, many of which are naturally occurring toxins and venoms. Sodium channels are critical to the conduction and propagation of action potentials along peripheral nerves. A select group of xenobiotics targeting the sodium channel are addressed in the final section of the article.

Acetylcholine

Similar to the neurotransmitters discussed earlier, acetylcholine is distributed throughout the brain and spinal cord. Unlike many other neurotransmitters, acetylcholine plays a major role in both the CNS and PNS. It is found in both sympathetic and parasympathetic presynaptic ganglia, parasympathetic postganglionic nerves, somatic motor neurons, and at most postganglionic sympathetically innervated sweat glands. Acetylcholine is synthesized by the enzyme choline acetyltransferase and is degraded within the synapse by acetylcholinesterase. A similar enzyme, pseudocholinesterase, is made in the liver and circulates in the plasma. It metabolizes some xenobiotics, like succinylcholine and cocaine, but does not play a large role in the metabolism of acetylcholine.

There are two major types of cholinergic receptors: nicotinic and muscarinic. Nicotinic receptors are ligand-gated ion channels. The receptors at the neuromuscular junction (NMJ nAchR) mediate sodium influx, stimulating depolarization of the endplate and propagation of an action potential down the muscle. Nicotinic receptors at other neuronal sites, both centrally and peripherally, mediate both sodium and calcium influx.[71] Although there are 5 different subtypes of muscarinic acetylcholine receptor, all are G-protein mediated.[73]

The central effects of acetylcholine are primarily mediated by muscarinic receptors because the majority of CNS nicotinic receptors reside in the spinal cord.[71] The central effects are usually accompanied by their corresponding peripheral effects.

Acetylcholine agonism can be produced by direct stimulation of acetylcholine receptors, or by inhibition of acetylcholinesterase (thereby increasing the amounts of acetylcholine within the nerve terminal). Excessive acetylcholine stimulation produces the classic cholinergic syndrome.[145] Central muscarinic effects include sedation, coma, extrapyramidal movement disorders, and seizures. Central nicotinic effects also include seizures. Peripheral muscarinic effects include excessive secretion at salivary, sweat, lacrimal, and bronchial glands, bronchoconstriction, nausea, vomiting, diarrhea, gastrointestinal cramping, urinary incontinence, and fecal incontinence, commonly coined the "SLUDGE" syndrome. Peripheral nicotinic effects include fasciculations, weakness, and flaccid paralysis. Weaponized nerve agents (eg, sarin and VX), organophosphate insecticides, and carbamate insecticides are the prototypical cholinergic agents.

Acetylcholine antagonism produces the collection of symptoms commonly referred to as the anticholinergic syndrome: hyperthermia, tachycardia, flushed skin, anhydrosis, mydriasis, hypoactive bowel sounds, urinary retention, delirium, agitation, picking movements, hallucinations, and coma. The mnemonic "hot as a hare, red as a beet, dry as a bone, blind as a bat, and mad as a hatter" summarizes the progression.[100] These symptoms are mediated predominately through inhibition at muscarinic sites, thus this syndrome is more precisely described as an antimuscarinic syndrome.[71] Hundreds of medications possess antimuscarinic properties, including atropine and other belladonna alkaloids, tricyclic antidepressants, phenothiazine antipsychotics, antiparkinsonian medications, and antihistamines. Natural causes of antimuscarinic poisoning include jimson weed (*Datura stramonium*), Deadly nightshade (*Atropa belladonna*), Angel's trumpet (*Cestrum nocturnum*), Henbane (*Hyoscyamus niger*), and Mandrake (*Mandragora officinarum*).[100]

The NMJ nAchR are a frequent target of xenobiotics that cause peripheral neurotoxic emergencies. The neurotoxic effects are produced in 1 of 3 ways: direct neuromuscular blockade, inhibition of acetylcholine release, or alteration of sodium channel function.

Snake Venom Neurotoxins

Neurotoxins comprise a small proportion of the complex mixture of enzymes, proteins, polypeptides, metals, and various other components in snake venom. The majority of snake neurotoxins cause a progressive generalized flaccid paralysis, initially affecting cranial nerves, with ptosis, ophthalmoplegia, dysarthria, dysphagia, and drooling, then progressing to generalized weakness and finally paralysis of the respiratory muscles.[146] The resultant respiratory paralysis is partially responsible for the estimated 125,000 deaths from snakebite each year.[146] Neuromuscular blockade at the NMJ nAchR is the mechanism by which these neurotoxic venoms exert their effects. Some venom neurotoxins, like those of coral snakes, cobras, and sea snakes, competitively block the NMJ nAchR.[147–150] These effects can be reversed by antivenom or with the administration of an anticholinesterase, such as neostigmine.[147,150] Venom from the Mojave rattlesnake (*Crotalus scutulatus*), and a few other *Crotalus* species, contains a different neurotoxin that inhibits the presynaptic release of acetylcholine from the neuromuscular junction.[148–150] Unless administered early, before the neurotoxin reaches the NMJ, antivenom is unlikely to be beneficial.[146,148] Acetylcholinesterase therapy is unhelpful in these instances.[150]

Tick Paralysis

Once attached a host, the mature female tick secretes a potent neurotoxin causing a slow, ascending, flaccid paralysis. More than 60 different species of tick are associated with tick paralysis. In the United States the most commonly associated species are the wood tick (*Dermacentor andersoni*) and the dog tick (*Dermacentor variabilis*).[151] Similar to the presynaptic snake toxins, the neurotoxin of tick paralysis inhibits the presynaptic release of acetylcholine at the NMJ, causing a symmetric ascending paralysis, and ultimately respiratory muscle failure.[151–153] Removal of the tick leads to gradual recovery, although in some Australian tick species (*Ixodes holocyclus*) recovery may be delayed.[151]

Botulism

Botulism poisoning (*botulus* is latin for sausage) has been well documented since the eighteenth century as a cause of descending flaccid paralysis.[154] Botulinum toxins (BOTOX) are exotoxins of the anaerobic spore-forming bacterium *Clostridium botulinum*. There are 8 different serotypes of *C botulinum*, which make 7 serologically distinct exotoxins (A-G).[155] Similar to tic paralysis and presynaptic snake neurotoxins, BOTOX blocks the release of acetylcholine presynaptically at the NMJ, initially leading to cranial nerve and bulbar symptoms (blurred vision, diplopia, dysarthria, dysphagia, or dysphonia), then progressing to an acute, symmetric, descending motor paralysis with little sensory or autonomic involvement.[154,156,157] BOTOX does not cross the blood-brain barrier, thus there are no central effects.[158]

Humans are exposed to BOTOX in a variety of ways. The most well known, food-borne botulism, occurs after ingestion of food contaminated with the preformed BOTOX. Wound botulism occurs when the spores of *C botulinum* in contaminated wounds germinate and produce BOTOX. The incidence of wound botulism is increasing in heroin addicts who subcutaneously inject black tar heroin ("skin popping").[157] Infant botulism occurs when spores are ingested and subsequently germinate in the infant's immature intestinal tract. Adult intestinal botulism occurs in adults with intestinal flora altered by antibiotic use and other gastrointestinal disorders. Weaponized, aerosolized BOTOX would cause inhalational botulism after release in a bioterrorism attack.[157,159]

Treatment includes vigilant supportive care with close observation for signs of respiratory weakness that might indicate the need for elective intubation and mechanical ventilation. Early antibiotics and surgical debridement are warranted in cases of wound botulism. Definitive treatment with botulinum antitoxin should be given to any patient with a clinical suspicion for botulism. Antitoxin neutralizes free BOTOX in the serum, thus it arrests the progression of symptoms but will not reverse those already present.[158] The standard botulinum antitoxin is horse-derived with antibodies against subtypes A, B, and E. It is obtained by contacting the local or state health department or the Centers for Disease Control and Prevention. BabyBIG is a human-derived immune globulin effective against subtypes A and B, used in the treatment of infant botulism.[157,158] The US Army possesses an antitoxin against all seven serotypes for use in the event of a bioterrorism event.[157,159]

Latrodectism

Widow spiders of the Genus *Latrodectus* are endemic worldwide. The black widow spider, *Latrodectus mactans*, is the most commonly recognized, due to the red hourglass-shaped markings on its ventral abdomen, but other *Latrodectus* species are also endemic in North America. Only the female spider is considered venomous because the smaller male's fangs are not large enough to penetrate human skin. The neurotoxin responsible for latrodectism, α-latrotoxin, facilitates calcium influx into the presynaptic neuron, stimulating massive release of acetylcholine at the neuromuscular junction.[160–162] α-Latrotoxin has similar effects at other peripheral and central acetylcholine and NE neurons as well.[161,163]

Predominant symptoms include muscle pain, spasms, and abdominal rigidity that on occasion has been mistaken for an acute surgical abdomen.[160,162,164] Accompanying symptoms include perspiration, restlessness, anxiety, nausea, vomiting, diarrhea, tachycardia, and hypertension.[162,163] Priapism, facies latrodectismica (facial grimacing), pavor mortis (fear of death), conjunctivitis, and compartment syndrome are less common.[163]

Treatment is supportive with local wound care, tetanus prophylaxis, and the liberal use of opioids and benzodiazepines for relief of pain, anxiety, and muscle spasms. Latrodectus antivenom is rapidly effective but its use is somewhat controversial, due to the very low risk of anaphylaxis and serum sickness. Development of a Fab fragment antivenom is currently under way. Alternative treatments, including calcium gluconate, methocarbamol, and dantrolene, have not proved to be effective.[165,166]

Glycine

Glycine is an inhibitory neurotransmitter found primarily in the spinal cord and lower brainstem, where it plays a large role in mediating motor and sensory reflex circuits. The glycine receptor is a ligand-gated chloride ion channel receptor similar in structure to the GABA$_A$ receptor.[167]

Strychnine

Strychnine is the natural alkaloid found in the dried seeds of the Southeast Asian tree, *Strychnos nux-vomica*.[168] Strychnine is used as a rodenticide, as a component of some traditional remedies, and as an occasional adulterant in street drugs such as amphetamines, heroin, and cocaine.[168–170] Strychnine is a competitive inhibitor at the glycine receptor. Glycine antagonism leads to uncontrolled muscular activity, initially causing heightened awareness, muscular spasms, and twitches, then progressing to generalized convulsions. The patient remains conscious, afraid, and in pain throughout the course.[168,170] Death is usually caused by respiratory arrest from respiratory muscle spasm. There is no known antidote; treatment is symptomatic and supportive. Benzodiazepines and barbiturates should be used liberally to control muscular spasms. If unsuccessful, nondepolarizing neuromuscular blockade with mechanical ventilation is required. Complications including hypoxia, aspiration, hyperthermia, rhabdomyolysis, and metabolic acidosis should be anticipated.

Tetanus

Tetanus (from the Greek word *tetanos*, to contract) has been known as a disease entity for over 20 centuries.[154] Under favorable anaerobic conditions, the bacillus *Clostridium tetani* produces tetanus toxin. The spores of *C tetani* are ubiquitous in the soil, but more prevalent in soil contaminated by the feces of animals.[171] These spores germinate in dirty wounds, leading to the production of tetanus toxin. Tetanus toxin inhibits the presynaptic release of GABA and glycine in a manner that closely parallels botulism.[154,156,157] There are 4 clinical types of tetanus.[157,171] Generalized tetanus is the most common, causing symptoms strikingly similar to those caused by strychnine. Opisthotonus and risus sardonicus are classically described in patients suffering from tetanus but can be seen in strychnine poisoning as well. With localized tetanus, rigidity and pain remain localized to the site of injury. Cephalic tetanus occurs with injuries to the head or neck and involves the lower cranial nerve musculature. Neonatal tetanus usually follows an umbilical stump infection and may initially present with failure to feed, inability to suck, and weakness. Treatment includes supportive care, wound management, antibiotics, active immunization with a tetanus toxoid–containing vaccine, and passive immunization with tetanus-specific immune globulin.[157,171] Similarly to strychnine, benzodiazepines are first-line agents for control of spasms. Nondepolarizing neuromuscular blockade and mechanical ventilation may be required in severe cases. A high suspicion for complications similar to those of strychnine should be maintained.

Sodium Channels

Just as nicotinic acetylcholine receptors mediate sodium influx through an ion channel, voltage-sensitive sodium ion channels mediate action potential propagation in skeletal muscle, nerve, and cardiac cells.[172] Slight alterations of sodium influx through these channels can easily produce detrimental consequences in membrane excitability. Several xenobiotics induce neurotoxic emergencies in this fashion, by altering sodium entry through these various voltage-sensitive sodium ion channels.

Ciguatera

Ciguatera poisoning is the most commonly reported marine food poisoning. The causative agent, ciguatoxin, is produced by the marine dinoflagellate, *Gambierdiscus toxicus*, and concentrates in the food chain as carnivorous fish eat the smaller herbivorous fish that ingest these dinoflagellates.[173] Humans ingest ciguatoxin when dining on large predatory reef fish including grouper, snapper, barracuda, amberjack, and sea bass.[158] Ciguatoxin binds to voltage-sensitive sodium channels, causing prolonged opening and excitation of skeletal, cardiac, and neuronal tissues.[158,174,175] Ciguatera poisoning leads to 4 categories of symptoms: gastrointestinal (nausea, vomiting, diarrhea), neuropathic (paresthesias, dysthesias, pruritus, diaphoresis, myalgias, arthralgias, weakness), cardiovascular (symptomatic bradycardia), and diffuse pain syndrome. Temperature allodynia (cold reversal, wherein cold items feel hot and possibly vice versa) and the sensation that the teeth are falling out are almost pathognomonic for ciguatera poisoning.[176] Treatment is largely supportive. Although mannitol has been recommended by some investigators, randomized controlled trials have failed to show benefit.[158,174,176]

Neurotoxic Shellfish Poisoning

Neurotoxic shellfish poisoning (NSP) is caused by brevetoxins, a family of toxins that, like ciguatera, open voltage-sensitive sodium channels.[173] The toxin is produced by the dinoflagellate *Kerenia brevis* (formerly *Gymnodinium breve*).[173,175] Brevetoxins are concentrated in filter-feeding shellfish (oysters, clams, coquinas, and other bivalve mollusks).[177] Symptoms are similar to the gastrointestinal and neuropathic symptoms of ciguatera poisoning, but typically resolve within 48 hours.[175] Treatment is supportive.

Poison Dart Frogs

Batrachotoxin is a potent sodium channel opener excreted from the skin of brightly colored *Phyllobates* frogs.[178] These frogs are commonly referred to as "poison dart frogs," presumably referring to the South American Indians' use of their secretions to poison the tips of blowdarts.

Paralytic Shellfish Poisoning

Paralytic shellfish poisoning (PSP) is the most common form of toxin-related disease associated with shellfish ingestion.[177] PSP toxins, saxitoxins, are produced by dinoflagellates of the genera *Alexandrium*. These toxins accumulate in filter-feeding shellfish (mussels, scallops, and clams) similar to NSP, but also have been found in the predators of shellfish, including crustaceans, gastropods, and fish.[175,177,179] Unlike the sodium channel openers discussed above, saxitoxins block voltage-gated sodium channels, preventing the generation of a proper action potential in nerves and muscles.[179] Symptoms include paresthesias, headache, nausea, vomiting, and diarrhea, followed by weakness, dysarthria, and dysphagia. In severe cases weakness progresses to neuromuscular paralysis and respiratory arrest.[175,177,179] Treatment is supportive.

Pufferfish Poisoning

Tetrodotoxin (TTX) is found in a variety of bony fish from the family *Tetraodontidae* including the pufferfish, toad fish, blowfish, balloon fish, and porcupine fish.[177] TTX is also found in a variety of other animals including certain mollusks, the horseshoe crab, the Californian newt, Costa Rican *Atelopus* frogs, and the blue-ringed octopus.[158,180] TTX poisoning is the most common cause of lethal food poisoning, especially in Japan, where pufferfish is consumed as a delicacy.[177] Similar to saxitoxins,

TTX blocks voltage-gated sodium channels, preventing nerve conduction.[158,175,177,180] The high fatality rate associated with TTX poisoning led to the development of a clinical grading system.[158,177] Grade 1 includes perioral numbness and paresthesias, with or without gastrointestinal symptoms. Grade 2 involves numbness of the tongue, face, and distal areas, early motor paralysis, uncoordination, and slurred speech. Grade 3 includes generalized flaccid paralysis, respiratory failure, aphonia, and fixed dilated pupils. In grade 4 patients suffer severe respiratory failure with hypoxia, hypotension, bradycardia, and cardiac arrhythmias.[158,177]

Treatment is supportive and focuses on ventilatory support. Lavage and activated charcoal should be considered in those presenting quickly after ingestion. Vasoactive pressor agents and mechanical ventilation may be necessary in moderate to severe cases.

SUMMARY

Acute neurotoxic emergencies manifest with a diverse array of clinical presentations that include drug-induced or toxin-induced seizures, acute excited mental status, acute depressed mental status, and a variety of PNS effects. Understanding the neurotransmitter interactions and pathophysiology of causative xenobiotics helps the provider anticipate the clinical effects of a particular exposure and directs focused therapeutic interventions.

REFERENCES

1. Stedman's medical dictionary. 25th edition. Baltimore(MD): Williams & Wilkins; 1990.
2. Thundiyil JG, Rowley F, Papa L, et al. Risk factors for complications of drug-induced seizures. J Med Toxicol 2011;7:16–23.
3. Thundiyil JG, Kearney TE, Olson KR. Evolving epidemiology of drug-induced seizures reported to a poison control center system. J Toxicol Clin Toxicol 2004;42(5):730.
4. Olson KR, Kearney TE, Dyer JE, et al. Seizures associated with poisoning and drug overdose. Am J Emerg Med 1994;12(3):392–5.
5. Sharma AN, Hoffman RJ. Toxin-related seizures. Emerg Med Clin North Am 2011;29(1):125–39.
6. Woolf AD, Erdman AR, Nelson LS, et al. Tricyclic antidepressant poisoning: an evidence-based consensus guideline for out-of-hospital management. Clin Toxicol (Phila) 2007;45(3):203–33.
7. Bebarta VS, Maddry J, Borys DJ, et al. Incidence of tricyclic antidepressant-like complications after cyclobenzaprine overdose. Am J Emerg Med 2010. [Epub ahead of print].
8. Bradberry SM, Thanacoody HK, Watt BE, et al. Management of the cardiovascular complications of tricyclic antidepressant poisoning: role of sodium bicarbonate. Toxicol Rev 2005;24(3):195–204.
9. Dhillon S, Yang LP, Curran MP. Spotlight on bupropion in major depressive disorder. CNS Drugs 2008;22(7):613–7.
10. Starr P, Klein-Schwartz W, Spiller H, et al. Incidence and onset of delayed seizures after overdoses of extended-release bupropion. Am J Emerg Med 2009;27(8):911–5.
11. Nelson LS, Erdman AR, Booze LL, et al. Selective serotonin reuptake inhibitor poisoning: an evidence-based consensus guideline for out-of-hospital management. Clin Toxicol (Phila) 2007;45(4):315–32.

12. Waring WS, Gray JA, Graham A. Predictive factors for generalized seizures after deliberate citalopram overdose. Br J Clin Pharmacol 2008;66(6):861–5.
13. Hayes BD, Klein-Schwartz W, Clark RF, et al. Comparison of toxicity of acute overdoses with citalopram and escitalopram. J Emerg Med 2010;39(1):44–8.
14. Yilmaz Z, Ceschi A, Rauber-Luthy C, et al. Escitalopram causes fewer seizures in human overdose than citalopram. Clin Toxicol (Phila) 2010;48(3):207–12.
15. Perucca E, Gram L, Avanzini G, et al. Antiepileptic drugs as a cause of worsening seizures. Epilepsia 1998;39(1):5–17.
16. Spiller HA, Carlisle RD. Status epilepticus after massive carbamazepine overdose. J Toxicol Clin Toxicol 2002;40(1):81–90.
17. Sullivan JB Jr, Rumack BH, Peterson RG. Acute carbamazepine toxicity resulting from overdose. Neurology 1981;31(5):621–4.
18. Guerrini R, Belmonte A, Parmeggiani L, et al. Myoclonic status epilepticus following high-dosage lamotrigine therapy. Brain Dev 1999;21(6):420–4.
19. Hasan M, Lerman-Sagie T, Lev D, et al. Recurrent absence status epilepticus (spike-and-wave stupor) associated with lamotrigine therapy. J Child Neurol 2006;21(9):807–9.
20. Trinka E, Dilitz E, Unterberger I, et al. Non convulsive status epilepticus after replacement of valproate with lamotrigine. J Neurol 2002;249(10):1417–22.
21. Dinnerstein E, Jobst BC, Williamson PD. Lamotrigine intoxication provoking status epilepticus in an adult with localization-related epilepsy. Arch Neurol 2007;64(9):1344–6.
22. Thundiyil JG, Anderson IB, Stewart PJ, et al. Lamotrigine-induced seizures in a child: case report and literature review. Clin Toxicol (Phila) 2007;45(2):169–72.
23. Anand JS, Chodorowski Z, Wisniewski M. Seizures induced by topiramate overdose. Clin Toxicol (Phila) 2007;45(2):197.
24. Wisniewski M, Lukasik-Glebocka M, Anand JS. Acute topiramate overdose—clinical manifestations. Clin Toxicol (Phila) 2009;47(4):317–20.
25. Jette N, Cappell J, VanPassel L, et al. Tiagabine-induced nonconvulsive status epilepticus in an adolescent without epilepsy. Neurology 2006;67(8):1514–5.
26. Kazzi ZN, Jones CC, Morgan BW. Seizures in a pediatric patient with a tiagabine overdose. J Med Toxicol 2006;2(4):160–2.
27. Ostrovskiy D, Spanaki MV, Morris GL 3rd. Tiagabine overdose can induce convulsive status epilepticus. Epilepsia 2002;43(7):773–4.
28. Devlin RJ, Henry JA. Clinical review: major consequences of illicit drug consumption. Crit Care 2008;12(1):202.
29. Paloucek FP, Rodvold KA. Evaluation of theophylline overdoses and toxicities. Ann Emerg Med 1988;17(2):135–44.
30. Shanti CM, Lucas CE. Cocaine and the critical care challenge. Crit Care Med 2003;31(6):1851–9.
31. Catravas JD, Waters IW. Acute cocaine intoxication in the conscious dog: studies on the mechanism of lethality. J Pharmacol Exp Ther 1981;217(2):350–6.
32. Gill JR, Hayes JA, deSouza IS, et al. Ecstasy (MDMA) deaths in New York City: a case series and review of the literature. J Forensic Sci 2002;47(1):121–6.
33. Kojima T, Une I, Yashiki M, et al. A fatal methamphetamine poisoning associated with hyperpyrexia. Forensic Sci Int 1984;24(1):87–93.
34. Patel MM, Belson MG, Longwater AB, et al. Methylenedioxymethamphetamine (ecstasy)-related hyperthermia. J Emerg Med 2005;29(4):451–4.
35. Young GP, Rores C, Murphy C, et al. Intravenous phenobarbital for alcohol withdrawal and convulsions. Ann Emerg Med 1987;16(8):847–50.

36. Hyser CL, Drake ME Jr. Status epilepticus after baclofen withdrawal. J Natl Med Assoc 1984;76(5):533, 537–8.
37. Kofler M, Arturo Leis A. Prolonged seizure activity after baclofen withdrawal. Neurology 1992;42(3 Pt 1):697–8.
38. Peng CT, Ger J, Yang CC, et al. Prolonged severe withdrawal symptoms after acute-on-chronic baclofen overdose. J Toxicol Clin Toxicol 1998;36(4):359–63.
39. Brust JC. Seizures and substance abuse: treatment considerations. Neurology 2006;67(12 Suppl 4):S45–8.
40. Grond S, Sablotzki A. Clinical pharmacology of tramadol. Clin Pharmacokinet 2004;43(13):879–923.
41. Jovanovic-Cupic V, Martinovic Z, Nesic N. Seizures associated with intoxication and abuse of tramadol. Clin Toxicol (Phila) 2006;44(2):143–6.
42. Shadnia S, Soltaninejad K, Heydari K, et al. Tramadol intoxication: a review of 114 cases. Hum Exp Toxicol 2008;27(3):201–5.
43. Spiller HA, Gorman SE, Villalobos D, et al. Prospective multicenter evaluation of tramadol exposure. J Toxicol Clin Toxicol 1997;35(4):361–4.
44. Afshari R, Ghooshkhanehee H. Tramadol overdose induced seizure, dramatic rise of CPK and acute renal failure. J Pak Med Assoc 2009;59(3):178.
45. Sansone RA, Sansone LA. Tramadol: seizures, serotonin syndrome, and coadministered antidepressants. Psychiatry (Edgmont) 2009;6(4):17–21.
46. Lawson AA, Northridge DB. Dextropropoxyphene overdose. Epidemiology, clinical presentation and management. Med Toxicol Adverse Drug Exp 1987;2(6):430–44.
47. Sloth Madsen P, Strom J, Reiz S, et al. Acute propoxyphene self-poisoning in 222 consecutive patients. Acta Anaesthesiol Scand 1984;28(6):661–5.
48. Stork CM, Redd JT, Fine K, et al. Propoxyphene-induced wide QRS complex dysrhythmia responsive to sodium bicarbonate—a case report. J Toxicol Clin Toxicol 1995;33(2):179–83.
49. Ramirez J, Innocenti F, Schuetz EG, et al. CYP2B6, CYP3A4, and CYP2C19 are responsible for the in vitro N-demethylation of meperidine in human liver microsomes. Drug Metab Dispos 2004;32(9):930–6.
50. Seifert CF, Kennedy S. Meperidine is alive and well in the new millennium: evaluation of meperidine usage patterns and frequency of adverse drug reactions. Pharmacotherapy 2004;24(6):776–83.
51. Maw G, Aitken P. Isoniazid overdose: a case series, literature review and survey of antidote availability. Clin Drug Investig 2003;23(7):479–85.
52. Vale JA, Kulig K. Position paper: gastric lavage. J Toxicol Clin Toxicol 2004;42(7):933–43.
53. Chyka PA, Seger D, Krenzelok EP, et al. Position paper: single-dose activated charcoal. Clin Toxicol (Phila) 2005;43(2):61–87.
54. Position paper: whole bowel irrigation. J Toxicol Clin Toxicol 2004;42(6):843–54.
55. Bryant SM, Weiselberg R, Metz J, et al. Should no bowel irrigation be a higher priority than whole bowel irrigation in the treatment of sustained-release ingestions? [abstract]. Clin Toxicol (Phila) 2008;47(7):638.
56. Position statement and practice guidelines on the use of multi-dose activated charcoal in the treatment of acute poisoning. American Academy of Clinical Toxicology; European Association of Poisons Centres and Clinical Toxicologists. J Toxicol Clin Toxicol 1999;37(6):731–51.
57. Proudfoot AT, Krenzelok EP, Vale JA. Position paper on urine alkalinization. J Toxicol Clin Toxicol 2004;42(1):1–26.

58. Wills B, Erickson T. Chemically induced seizures. Clin Lab Med 2006;26(1): 185–209, ix.

59. Nolop KB, Natow A. Unprecedented sedative requirements during delirium tremens. Crit Care Med 1985;13(4):246–7.

60. Woo E, Greenblatt DJ. Massive benzodiazepine requirements during acute alcohol withdrawal. Am J Psychiatry 1979;136(6):821–3.

61. Coomes TR, Smith SW. Successful use of propofol in refractory delirium tremens. Ann Emerg Med 1997;30(6):825–8.

62. McCowan C, Marik P. Refractory delirium tremens treated with propofol: a case series. Crit Care Med 2000;28(6):1781–4.

63. Claassen J, Hirsch LJ, Emerson RG, et al. Treatment of refractory status epilepticus with pentobarbital, propofol, or midazolam: a systematic review. Epilepsia 2002;43(2):146–53.

64. Rossetti AO, Reichhart MD, Schaller MD, et al. Propofol treatment of refractory status epilepticus: a study of 31 episodes. Epilepsia 2004;45(7):757–63.

65. Shah AS, Eddleston M. Should phenytoin or barbiturates be used as second-line anticonvulsant therapy for toxicological seizures? Clin Toxicol (Phila) 2010;48(8):800–5.

66. Bazil CW, Pedley TA. Clinical pharmacology of antiepileptic drugs. Clin Neuropharmacol 2003;26(1):38–52.

67. Tutka P, Mroz T, Klucha K, et al. Bupropion-induced convulsions: preclinical evaluation of antiepileptic drugs. Epilepsy Res 2005;64(1/2):13–22.

68. Brent J, Vo N, Kulig K, et al. Reversal of prolonged isoniazid-induced coma by pyridoxine. Arch Intern Med 1990;150(8):1751–3.

69. Shannon M, McElroy EA, Liebelt EL. Toxic seizures in children: case scenarios and treatment strategies. Pediatr Emerg Care 2003;19(3):206–10.

70. Uusi-Oukari M, Korpi ER. Regulation of GABA(A) receptor subunit expression by pharmacological agents. Pharmacol Rev 2010;62(1):97–135.

71. Curry SC, Mills KC, Ruha AM, et al. Neurotransmitters and neuromodulators. In: Nelson LS, Lewin NA, Howland MA, et al, editors. Goldfrank's toxicologic emergencies. 9th edition. New York: McGraw-Hill Companies; 2011. p. 189–220.

72. Bormann J. The 'ABC' of GABA receptors. Trends Pharmacol Sci 2000;21(1): 16–9.

73. Akhtar J, Rittenberger JC. Clinical neurotoxicology. In: Shannon MW, Borron SW, Burns MJ, editors. Haddad and Winchester's clinical management of poisoning and drug overdose. 4th edition. Philadelphia: Elsevier; 2007. p. 191–207.

74. Korpi ER, Mattila MJ, Wisden W, et al. GABA(A)-receptor subtypes: clinical efficacy and selectivity of benzodiazepine site ligands. Ann Med 1997;29(4): 275–82.

75. Luddens H, Korpi ER, Seeburg PH. GABA_A/benzodiazepine receptor heterogeneity: neurophysiological implications. Neuropharmacology 1995;34(3):245–54.

76. Olsen RW, Li GD. GABA(A) receptors as molecular targets of general anesthetics: identification of binding sites provides clues to allosteric modulation. Can J Anaesth 2011;58(2):206–15.

77. Halpern JH. Hallucinogens and dissociative agents naturally growing in the United States. Pharmacol Ther 2004;102(2):131–8.

78. Shirley KW, Kothare S, Piatt JH Jr, et al. Intrathecal baclofen overdose and withdrawal. Pediatr Emerg Care 2006;22(4):258–61.

79. Chateauvieux S, Morceau F, Dicato M, et al. Molecular and therapeutic potential and toxicity of valproic acid. J Biomed Biotechnol 2010;2010:479364.

80. Mesdjian E, Ciesielski L, Valli M, et al. Sodium valproate: kinetic profile and effects on GABA levels in various brain areas of the rat. Prog Neuropsychopharmacol Biol Psychiatry 1982;6(3):223–33.
81. Urban MO, Ren K, Park KT, et al. Comparison of the antinociceptive profiles of gabapentin and 3-methylgabapentin in rat models of acute and persistent pain: implications for mechanism of action. J Pharmacol Exp Ther 2005;313(3):1209–16.
82. Sarup A, Larsson OM, Schousboe A. GABA transporters and GABA-transaminase as drug targets. Curr Drug Targets CNS Neurol Disord 2003;2(4):269–77.
83. McNamara JO. Pharmacotherapy of the epilepsies. In: Brunton LL, Lazo JS, Parker KL, editors. Goodman & Gillman's the pharmacological basis of therapeutics. 11th edition. New York: Mc-Graw Hill; 2005. p. 501–25.
84. Ngo AS, Anthony CR, Samuel M, et al. Should a benzodiazepine antagonist be used in unconscious patients presenting to the emergency department? Resuscitation 2007;74(1):27–37.
85. Seger DL. Flumazenil—treatment or toxin. J Toxicol Clin Toxicol 2004;42(2): 209–16.
86. Nemeth Z, Kun B, Demetrovics Z. The involvement of gamma-hydroxybutyrate in reported sexual assaults: a systematic review. J Psychopharmacol 2010; 24(9):1281–7.
87. Carter LP, Koek W, France CP. Behavioral analyses of GHB: receptor mechanisms. Pharmacol Ther 2009;121(1):100–14.
88. Maitre M. The gamma-hydroxybutyrate signalling system in brain: organization and functional implications. Prog Neurobiol 1997;51(3):337–61.
89. Wong CG, Gibson KM, Snead OC 3rd. From the street to the brain: neurobiology of the recreational drug gamma-hydroxybutyric acid. Trends Pharmacol Sci 2004;25(1):29–34.
90. Li J, Stokes SA, Woeckener A. A tale of novel intoxication: a review of the effects of gamma-hydroxybutyric acid with recommendations for management. Ann Emerg Med 1998;31(6):729–36.
91. Liechti ME, Kunz I, Greminger P, et al. Clinical features of gamma-hydroxybutyrate and gamma-butyrolactone toxicity and concomitant drug and alcohol use. Drug Alcohol Depend 2006;81(3):323–6.
92. Zvosec DL, Smith SW, McCutcheon JR, et al. Adverse events, including death, associated with the use of 1,4-butanediol. N Engl J Med 2001;344(2):87–94.
93. Shannon M, Quang LS. Gamma-hydroxybutyrate, gamma-butyrolactone, and 1,4-butanediol: a case report and review of the literature. Pediatr Emerg Care 2000;16(6):435–40.
94. Van Sassenbroeck DK, De Neve N, De Paepe P, et al. Abrupt awakening phenomenon associated with gamma-hydroxybutyrate use: a case series. Clin Toxicol (Phila) 2007;45(5):533–8.
95. Farmer BM. Gamma-hydroxybutyric acid. In: Nelson LS, Lewin NA, Howland MA, et al, editors. Goldfrank's toxicologic emergencies. 9th edition. New York: McGraw Hill; 2011. p. 1151–6.
96. Quang LS. GHB and related compounds. In: Shannon MW, Borron SW, Burns MJ, editors. Haddad and Winchester's clinical management of poisoning and drug overdose. 4th edition. Philadelphia: Elsevier; 2007. p. 803–23.
97. LeTourneau JL, Hagg DS, Smith SM. Baclofen and gamma-hydroxybutyrate withdrawal. Neurocrit Care 2008;8(3):430–3.
98. Trescot AM, Datta S, Lee M, et al. Opioid pharmacology. Pain Physician 2008; 11(Suppl 2):S133–53.

99. Dietis N, Guerrini R, Calo G, et al. Simultaneous targeting of multiple opioid receptors: a strategy to improve side-effect profile. Br J Anaesth 2009;103(1): 38–49.

100. Meehan TJ, Bryant SM, Aks SE. Drugs of abuse: the highs and lows of altered mental states in the emergency department. Emerg Med Clin North Am 2010; 28(3):663–82.

101. Dahan A, Aarts L, Smith TW. Incidence, reversal, and prevention of opioid-induced respiratory depression. Anesthesiology 2010;112(1):226–38.

102. Vardakou I, Pistos C, Spiliopoulou C. Spice drugs as a new trend: mode of action, identification and legislation. Toxicol Lett 2010;197(3):157–62.

103. Schneir AB, Cullen J, Ly BT. "Spice" girls: synthetic cannabinoid intoxication. J Emerg Med 2011;40(3):296–9.

104. Elkashef A, Vocci F, Huestis M, et al. Marijuana neurobiology and treatment. Subst Abus 2008;29(3):17–29.

105. Felder CC, Glass M. Cannabinoid receptors and their endogenous agonists. Annu Rev Pharmacol Toxicol 1998;38:179–200.

106. McPartland JM. The endocannabinoid system: an osteopathic perspective. J Am Osteopath Assoc 2008;108(10):586–600.

107. Ashton CH. Pharmacology and effects of cannabis: a brief review. Br J Psychiatry 2001;178:101–6.

108. Iversen L. Cannabis and the brain. Brain 2003;126(Pt 6):1252–70.

109. Campbell FA, Tramer MR, Carroll D, et al. Are cannabinoids an effective and safe treatment option in the management of pain? A qualitative systematic review. BMJ 2001;323(7303):13–6.

110. Johns A. Psychiatric effects of cannabis. Br J Psychiatry 2001;178:116–22.

111. Every-Palmer S. Synthetic cannabinoid JWH-018 and psychosis: an explorative study. Drug Alcohol Depend 2011. [Epub ahead of print].

112. Zimmermann US, Winkelmann PR, Pilhatsch M, et al. Withdrawal phenomena and dependence syndrome after the consumption of "spice gold". Dtsch Arztebl Int 2009;106(27):464–7.

113. Insel PA. Seminars in medicine of the Beth Israel Hospital, Boston. Adrenergic receptors—evolving concepts and clinical implications. N Engl J Med 1996; 334(9):580–5.

114. Beaulieu JM, Gainetdinov RR. The physiology, signaling, and pharmacology of dopamine receptors. Pharmacol Rev 2011;63(1):182–217.

115. Millan MJ, Marin P, Bockaert J, et al. Signaling at G-protein-coupled serotonin receptors: recent advances and future research directions. Trends Pharmacol Sci 2008;29(9):454–64.

116. Green AR, Mechan AO, Elliott JM, et al. The pharmacology and clinical pharmacology of 3,4-methylenedioxymethamphetamine (MDMA, "ecstasy"). Pharmacol Rev 2003;55(3):463–508.

117. Sulzer D, Sonders MS, Poulsen NW, et al. Mechanisms of neurotransmitter release by amphetamines: a review. Prog Neurobiol 2005;75(6):406–33.

118. Aghajanian GK, Marek GJ. Serotonin and hallucinogens. Neuropsychopharmacology 1999;21(Suppl 2):16S–23S.

119. DEA. Methylenedioxypyrovalerone (MDPV). Drugs and chemicals of concern. 2011. Available at: http://www.deadiversion.usdoj.gov/drugs_concern/mdpv. pdf. Accessed March 26, 2011.

120. ACMD. Consideration of the cathinones. Advisory council on the misuse of drugs. 2010. Available at: http://www.namsdl.org/documents/ACMDCathinonesReport. pdf. Accessed March 26, 2011.

121. Schwartz BG, Rezkalla S, Kloner RA. Cardiovascular effects of cocaine. Circulation 2010;122(24):2558–69.

122. Smith JA, Mo Q, Guo H, et al. Cocaine increases extraneuronal levels of aspartate and glutamate in the nucleus accumbens. Brain Res 1995;683(2):264–9.

123. Guidelines 2000 for cardiopulmonary resuscitation and emergency cardiovascular care. Part 8: advanced challenges in resuscitation: section 2: toxicology in ECC. The American Heart Association in collaboration with the International Liaison Committee on Resuscitation. Circulation 2000;102(Suppl 8):I223–8.

124. Albertson TE, Dawson A, de Latorre F, et al. TOX-ACLS: toxicologic-oriented advanced cardiac life support. Ann Emerg Med 2001;37(Suppl 4):S78–90.

125. Lange RA, Cigarroa RG, Flores ED, et al. Potentiation of cocaine-induced coronary vasoconstriction by beta-adrenergic blockade. Ann Intern Med 1990;112(12):897–903.

126. Boyer EW, Shannon M. The serotonin syndrome. N Engl J Med 2005;352(11):1112–20.

127. Juurlink DN. Antipsychotics. In: Nelson LS, Lewin NA, Howland MA, et al, editors. Goldfrank's toxicologic emergencies. 9th edition. New York: McGraw Hill; 2011. p. 1103–15.

128. Levine M, Burns MJ. Antipsychotic agents. In: Shannon MW, Borron SW, Burns MJ, editors. Haddad and Winchester's clinical management of poisoning and drug overdose. 4th edition. Philadelphia: Elsevier; 2007. p. 703–20.

129. Adnet P, Lestavel P, Krivosic-Horber R. Neuroleptic malignant syndrome. Br J Anaesth 2000;85(1):129–35.

130. Strawn JR, Keck PE Jr, Caroff SN. Neuroleptic malignant syndrome. Am J Psychiatry 2007;164(6):870–6.

131. Reulbach U, Dutsch C, Biermann T, et al. Managing an effective treatment for neuroleptic malignant syndrome. Crit Care 2007;11(1):R4.

132. Ener RA, Meglathery SB, Van Decker WA, et al. Serotonin syndrome and other serotonergic disorders. Pain Med 2003;4(1):63–74.

133. Birmes P, Coppin D, Schmitt L, et al. Serotonin syndrome: a brief review. CMAJ 2003;168(11):1439–42.

134. Isbister GK, Buckley NA. The pathophysiology of serotonin toxicity in animals and humans: implications for diagnosis and treatment. Clin Neuropharmacol 2005;28(5):205–14.

135. Radomski JW, Dursun SM, Reveley MA, et al. An exploratory approach to the serotonin syndrome: an update of clinical phenomenology and revised diagnostic criteria. Med Hypotheses 2000;55(3):218–24.

136. Javitt DC. Glutamate as a therapeutic target in psychiatric disorders. Mol Psychiatry 2004;9(11):984–97, 979.

137. Kew JN, Kemp JA. Ionotropic and metabotropic glutamate receptor structure and pharmacology. Psychopharmacology (Berl) 2005;179(1):4–29.

138. Mori H, Mishina M. Structure and function of the NMDA receptor channel. Neuropharmacology 1995;34(10):1219–37.

139. Weiner AL, Vieira L, McKay CA, et al. Ketamine abusers presenting to the emergency department: a case series. J Emerg Med 2000;18(4):447–51.

140. Bahn EL, Holt KR. Procedural sedation and analgesia: a review and new concepts. Emerg Med Clin North Am 2005;23(2):503–17.

141. Reich DL, Silvay G. Ketamine: an update on the first twenty-five years of clinical experience. Can J Anaesth 1989;36(2):186–97.

142. Liang IE, Boyer EW. Dissociative agents: phencyclidine, ketamine and dextromethorphan. In: Shannon MW, Borron SW, Burns MJ, editors. Haddad and

Winchester's clinical management of poisoning and drug overdose. 4th edition. Philadelphia: Elsevier; 2007. p. 773–9.

143. Jeffery B, Barlow T, Moizer K, et al. Amnesic shellfish poison. Food Chem Toxicol 2004;42(4):545–57.

144. Lefebvre KA, Robertson A. Domoic acid and human exposure risks: a review. Toxicon 2010;56(2):218–30.

145. Sidell FR, Borak J. Chemical warfare agents: II. Nerve agents. Ann Emerg Med 1992;21(7):865–71.

146. White J, Warrell D, Eddleston M, et al. Clinical toxinology—where are we now? J Toxicol Clin Toxicol 2003;41(3):263–76.

147. Khandelwal G, Katz KD, Brooks DE, et al. Naja Kaouthia: two cases of Asiatic cobra envenomations. J Emerg Med 2007;32(2):171–4.

148. Prasarnpun S, Walsh J, Awad SS, et al. Envenoming bites by kraits: the biological basis of treatment-resistant neuromuscular paralysis. Brain 2005;128(Pt 12): 2987–96.

149. Rowan EG. What does beta-bungarotoxin do at the neuromuscular junction? Toxicon 2001;39(1):107–18.

150. Sanmuganathan PS. Myasthenic syndrome of snake envenomation: a clinical and neurophysiological study. Postgrad Med J 1998;74(876):596–9.

151. Edlow JA, McGillicuddy DC. Tick paralysis. Infect Dis Clin North Am 2008;22(3): 397–413, vii.

152. Felz MW, Smith CD, Swift TR. A six-year-old girl with tick paralysis. N Engl J Med 2000;342(2):90–4.

153. Greenstein P. Tick paralysis. Med Clin North Am 2002;86(2):441–6.

154. Humeau Y, Doussau F, Grant NJ, et al. How botulinum and tetanus neurotoxins block neurotransmitter release. Biochimie 2000;82(5):427–46.

155. Klein AW. Complications and adverse reactions with the use of botulinum toxin. Semin Cutan Med Surg 2001;20(2):109–20.

156. Caleo M, Schiavo G. Central effects of tetanus and botulinum neurotoxins. Toxicon 2009;54(5):593–9.

157. Goonetilleke A, Harris JB. Clostridial neurotoxins. J Neurol Neurosurg Psychiatry 2004;75(Suppl 3):iii35–9.

158. Lawrence DT, Dobmeier SG, Bechtel LK, et al. Food poisoning [abstract ix]. Emerg Med Clin North Am 2007;25(2):357–73.

159. Arnon SS, Schechter R, Inglesby TV, et al. Botulinum toxin as a biological weapon: medical and public health management. JAMA 2001;285(8):1059–70.

160. Handel CC, Izquierdo LA, Curet LB. Black widow spider (Latrodectus mactans) bite during pregnancy. West J Med 1994;160(3):261–2.

161. Ushkaryov YA, Volynski KE, Ashton AC. The multiple actions of black widow spider toxins and their selective use in neurosecretion studies. Toxicon 2004; 43(5):527–42.

162. Vetter RS, Isbister GK. Medical aspects of spider bites. Annu Rev Entomol 2008; 53:409–29.

163. Graudins A. Spiders. In: Shannon MW, Borron SW, Burns MJ, editors. Haddad and Winchester's clinical management of poisoning and drug overdose. 4th edition. Philadelphia: Elsevier; 2007. p. 433–9.

164. Hahn I. Arthropods. In: Nelson LS, Lewin NA, Howland MA, et al, editors. Goldfrank's toxicologic emergencies. 9th edition. New York: McGraw Hill; 2011. p. 1561–81.

165. Daly FF, Hill RE, Bogdan GM, et al. Neutralization of *Latrodectus mactans* and *L. hesperus* venom by redback spider (*L. hasseltii*) antivenom. J Toxicol Clin Toxicol 2001;39(2):119–23.

166. Isbister GK, Graudins A, White J, et al. Antivenom treatment in arachnidism. J Toxicol Clin Toxicol 2003;41(3):291–300.

167. Webb TI, Lynch JW. Molecular pharmacology of the glycine receptor chloride channel. Curr Pharm Des 2007;13(23):2350–67.

168. Makarovsky I, Markel G, Hoffman A, et al. Strychnine—a killer from the past. Isr Med Assoc J 2008;10(2):142–5.

169. Chan TY. Herbal medicine causing likely strychnine poisoning. Hum Exp Toxicol 2002;21(8):467–8.

170. Wood D, Webster E, Martinez D, et al. Case report: survival after deliberate strychnine self-poisoning, with toxicokinetic data. Crit Care 2002;6(5):456–9.

171. Afshar M, Raju M, Ansell D, et al. Narrative review: tetanus—a health threat after natural disasters in developing countries. Ann Intern Med 2011;154(5):329–35.

172. Wang SY, Wang GK. Voltage-gated sodium channels as primary targets of diverse lipid-soluble neurotoxins. Cell Signal 2003;15(2):151–9.

173. Wang DZ. Neurotoxins from marine dinoflagellates: a brief review. Mar Drugs 2008;6(2):349–71.

174. Purcell CE, Capra MF, Cameron J. Action of mannitol in ciguatoxin-intoxicated rats. Toxicon 1999;37(1):67–76.

175. Sobel J, Painter J. Illnesses caused by marine toxins. Clin Infect Dis 2005;41(9):1290–6.

176. Schnorf H, Taurarii M, Cundy T. Ciguatera fish poisoning: a double-blind randomized trial of mannitol therapy. Neurology 2002;58(6):873–80.

177. Isbister GK. Marine envenomation and poisoning. In: Dart RC, editor. Medical toxicology. 3rd edition. Philadelphia: Lippincott Williams & Wilkins; 2004. p. 1621–44.

178. Bosmans F, Maertens C, Verdonck F, et al. The poison dart frog's batrachotoxin modulates Nav1.8. FEBS Lett 2004;577(1–2):245–8.

179. Araoz R, Molgo J, Tandeau de Marsac N. Neurotoxic cyanobacterial toxins. Toxicon 2010;56(5):813–28.

180. How CK, Chern CH, Huang YC, et al. Tetrodotoxin poisoning. Am J Emerg Med 2003;21(1):51–4.

Antidepressant Overdose–induced Seizures

Bryan S. Judge, MD[a,b,c],*, Landen L. Rentmeester, MD[a,b]

KEYWORDS

- Antidepressants • Overdose • Seizures
- Deliberate self-poisoning

Human exposure to antidepressants in the United States has rapidly escalated in recent years. Although millions of Americans therapeutically take this class of neuro-active drugs on a daily basis,[1] exposures can also occur after an accidental ingestion or from an intentional overdose. In 2009, antidepressants as a class ranked seventh (n = 102,792) among substance categories most frequently involved in human exposures reported to the National Poison Data System (NPDS).[2] Regardless of the intent of the exposure, antidepressants can result in seizures.[3] Although seizures associated with the therapeutic use of antidepressants are infrequent, their risk after overdose is much greater.[4] Furthermore, antidepressant overdose–induced seizures can generate dilemmas for the clinician such as treating status epilepticus,[5] or determining the need for, and duration of, inpatient monitoring.

Because antidepressant use among patients is common, and because they are frequently involved in intentional and unintentional overdoses, it would benefit practitioners to (1) recognize the seizure propensity associated with various antidepressants, (2) understand the mechanism(s) underlying antidepressant overdose–induced seizures, and (3) be familiar with treatment strategies for patients who have experienced an antidepressant overdose–induced seizure. Therefore, the focus of this review is threefold. First, the classes of antidepressants, their pharmacologic properties, along with some of the proposed mechanism(s) for seizures triggered by antidepressants in overdose, are discussed briefly. Second, pertinent evidence for antidepressant

---

The authors have no conflicts, financial or otherwise, to disclose.

[a] Grand Rapids Medical Education Partners/Michigan State University Emergency Medicine Residency, 100 Michigan NE, MC 49, Grand Rapids, MI 49403, USA

[b] Division of Emergency Medicine, Michigan State University College of Human Medicine, 15 Michigan Street NE, Suite 425, Grand Rapids, MI 49503, USA

[c] Spectrum Health-Toxicology Services, 1900 Wealthy Street SE, Suite 255, Grand Rapids, MI 49506, USA

* Corresponding author. Spectrum Health-Toxicology Services, 1900 Wealthy Street SE, Suite 255, Grand Rapids, MI 49506.

E-mail address: bryan.judge@spectrum-health.org

Neurol Clin 29 (2011) 565–580

doi:10.1016/j.ncl.2011.05.003

0733-8619/11/$ – see front matter © 2011 Elsevier Inc. All rights reserved.

overdose–induced seizures is examined and, after careful scrutiny of this evidence, antidepressants are ranked as high risk (seizure incidence >10% after overdose), intermediate risk (seizure incidence 5%–10% after overdose), or low risk (seizure incidence <5% after overdose) for seizure potential. In addition, management strategies are provided for patients who have intentionally or unintentionally overdosed on an antidepressant, or who have experienced an antidepressant overdose–induced seizure.

PATHOPHYSIOLOGY OF SEIZURE ACTIVITY

Before discussing the various antidepressant classes and the mechanism(s) that may be responsible for antidepressant overdose–induced seizures, it is paramount to briefly review the pathways by which seizures can be triggered. In general, neuronal excitation results from an influx of sodium or diminishment of either chloride conduction or potassium efflux through ion channels. Conversely, neuronal inhibition occurs after a decrease in sodium influx or augmentation of either chloride conduction or potassium efflux through ion channels. When there is gross imbalance between neuronal excitation and inhibition, electrical activity within the central nervous system (CNS) becomes frenzied, and seizures ensue.[6]

There are numerous neurochemical pathways recognized for triggering seizures. Drugs that antagonize adenosine (A$_1$), histamine (H$_1$), and γ-aminobutyric acid (GABA) receptors can result in seizures,[7–9] and substances that stimulate cholinergic and glutamatergic receptors can trigger seizures.[10,11] The role of sodium channels in the development and treatment of seizures is complex; although drugs that block sodium channels are often used to prevent seizures (eg, phenytoin), this same mechanism can cause seizures such as those seen with excessive doses of lidocaine.[12] This exemplifies the complex nature underlying the cause and treatment of seizures. Numerous metabolic disturbances can produce seizures: hypocalcemia, hypoglycemia, hyperglycemia, hypomagnesemia, and hyponatremia.[6] Contrary to prior dogma, a solid body of evidence now supports the concept that the noradrenergic and serotonergic effects of antidepressants are anticonvulsant with therapeutic doses, whereas larger doses, such as those that occur with supratherapeutic exposure or an intentional overdose, activate other neurochemical pathways that can culminate in seizures.[13,14]

CLASSIFICATION OF ANTIDEPRESSANTS
Monoamine Oxidase Inhibitors (Isocarboxazid, Moclobemide, Phenelzine, Selegiline, Tranylcypromine)

Monoamine oxidase inhibitors (MAOI) were the first drugs used to treat depression, and were once considered first-line pharmacologic therapy. There are several drugs in this class; however, only a few are used today in the United States for the treatment of refractory depression; these include isocarboxazid, phenelzine, selegiline (transdermal system), and tranylcypromine.[15] Currently, moclobemide is approved as an antidepressant in several countries worldwide but has not been approved for use in the United States.[16]

The primary pharmacologic mechanism by which MAOIs work is the inhibition of the enzyme monoamine oxidase located on the outer mitochondrial membrane of neurons.[17] Consequently, the breakdown of the biogenic amines dopamine, norepinephrine, and serotonin is prevented, thereby increasing the concentration of these neurotransmitters available for reuptake, storage, and subsequent release by neurons.[18] Isocarboxazid, phenelzine, and tranylcypromine are irreversible and nonselective MAOIs; selegiline irreversibly and selectively inhibits monoamine oxidase B; and moclobemide reversibly and selectively inhibits monoamine oxidase A.[16]

Although moclobemide may possess anticonvulsant properties,[19] there is potential for CNS excitation with overdose of the hydrazine derivatives isocarboxazid and phenelzine, and the amphetamine derivative tranylcypromine. Hydrazine derivatives including the antitubercular agent isoniazid diminish the synthesis of GABA in the CNS by antagonizing pyridoxine.[20] The net effect is loss of the normal neural inhibition mediated by GABA, resulting in seizures that are refractory unless treated with pyridoxine. In addition, isocarboxazid and tranylcypromine have been shown to block $GABA_A$ receptors in an animal model[21] and MAOIs may augment CNS excitation by increasing concentrations of neuronal glutamic acid.[22]

Cyclic Antidepressants (Tertiary Amines: Amitriptyline, Clomipramine, Doxepin, Imipramine, Trimipramine. Secondary Amines: Desipramine, Nortriptyline, Protriptyline. Other: Amoxapine, Maprotiline)

Although there has been a substantial decline in the number of people treated with cyclic antidepressants (CAs) in the United States,[1] poisoning and death from the intentional ingestions of this class of antidepressants remains problematic. In 2009, CAs comprised 11.6% (n = 11,873) of human exposures to antidepressants registered with the NPDS, and this substance category tied for 10th place among other substance categories associated with the largest number of fatalities.[2] Cyclic antidepressants can be classified into tertiary amines, which include amitriptyline, clomipramine, doxepin, imipramine, and trimipramine, and secondary amines, which include desipramine, nortriptyline, and protriptyline. Structurally, secondary amines differ from tertiary amines in that they lack a methyl group on the terminal nitrogen of their side chains. The dibenzoxapine CA amoxapine and the tetracyclic antidepressant maprotiline are discussed separately later.

The CAs have a multitude of pharmacologic actions. Their therapeutic effect is primarily mediated through the inhibition of the reuptake of the biogenic amines norepinephrine and serotonin.[23] Toxicity associated with CAs is caused by antagonism of α_1-adrenergic, H_1 histamine, and muscarinic receptors; blockade of cardiac ion channels (Na^+ and K^+); and interference with chloride conductance through GABA Cl^- ionophores.[6,24] Each drug within this class shows variability in these pharmacologic mechanisms of action and their toxic effects. Seizures after a CA overdose are believed to occur secondary to their interference with the influx of chloride through GABA Cl^- channels; these drugs bind to the picrotoxin site on the GABA-chloride complex,[21] but other potential mechanisms include an inhibitory effect on G-protein-activated inwardly rectifying K^+ (GIRK) channels or antagonism of H_1 receptors.[13]

Amoxapine

Introduced in 1980, amoxapine was initially promoted as having a faster onset of antidepressant effects compared with other available CAs.[25] Amoxapine inhibits the reuptake of norepinephrine, moderately antagonizes α_1-adrenergic and D_2 dopamine receptors, and weakly blocks H_1 receptors.[24] Seizure activity is one of the most common adverse reactions reported with amoxapine. Data from the World Health Organization's adverse drug reaction database from 1968 to 2006 noted 121 cases of convulsions out of 1384 reported adverse reactions.[26] Although these data are limited because the total number of patients taking amoxapine in this time period is not known, the percentage of adverse reactions reported as seizures for amoxapine (8.74%) was second only to maprotiline (14.43%) among the CAs. As with other antidepressants, the precise mechanism behind the proconvulsant effect of amoxapine is not fully understood.

Maprotiline

Similar to amoxapine, maprotiline inhibits the reuptake of norepinephrine, and moderately antagonizes α_1-adrenergic receptors, but differs in that it strongly blocks H_1 receptors and weakly antagonizes D_2 and muscarinic receptors.[24] This CA was initially believed to have a safer side effect profile compared with other CAs. However, even with therapeutic use, seizures have been an issue, and the risk for seizures seems to be dose-dependent.[27] One retrospective study found a seizure rate of 15.6% in patients taking between 75 and 300 mg daily.[28] Although it is uncertain what mechanism(s) are responsible for maprotiline-induced seizures, two possibilities include the inhibitory effect that maprotiline exerts on GIRK channels and antagonism of H_1 receptors.[13]

Selective Serotonin Reuptake Inhibitors (Citalopram, Escitalopram, Fluoxetine, Fluvoxamine, Paroxetine, Sertraline)

Because of their tolerability and relative safety in overdose compared with CAs, selective serotonin reuptake inhibitors (SSRIs) have been the preferred class of antidepressants to treat depression since the 1990s.[29] Several SSRIs are available, including citalopram, escitalopram, fluoxetine, fluvoxamine, paroxetine, and sertraline. The pharmacologic mechanism of action for this class of antidepressants is the selective inhibition of serotonin reuptake at the neuronal synapse. In addition, drugs in this class have many other pharmacologic properties: citalopram, fluoxetine, paroxetine, and sertraline also exhibit antimuscarinic activity; dopamine reuptake is inhibited by paroxetine and sertraline; and sertraline weakly antagonizes α-adrenergic receptors.[17] Despite their relative receptor selectivity, SSRIs can be proconvulsant in the setting of an overdose.[30] How this occurs is still not known.

Overdose of SSRIs can cause serotonin syndrome. Although seizures may be more likely to occur in this setting, not all SSRI overdose–induced seizures result from serotonin syndrome.[30,31] This class of antidepressants can also cause hyponatremia brought on by the syndrome of inappropriate antidiuretic hormone secretion (SIADH)[32] and this mechanism has caused seizures with therapeutic use of paroxetine[33] and could potentially cause a seizure after SSRI overdose. Inhibition of glycine receptors could also play a role in SSRI overdose–induced seizures.[34] Special mention should be made of citalopram, which is a racemic mixture, containing both R and S enantiomers, whereas escitalopram contains the S enantiomer.[35] Some investigators have suggested that the R enantiomer of citalopram is responsible for the more serious toxic effects (QTc prolongation and seizures) of this drug,[35] whereas others have speculated that seizures induced by citalopram may occur from inhibition of GIRK channels.[13]

Atypical Antidepressants (Bupropion, Duloxetine, Mirtazapine, Reboxetine, Trazodone, Venlafaxine)

Atypical antidepressants consist of those drugs not belonging to the MAOI, SSRI, or CA classes. These drugs are new, share structural similarity with the SSRIs, and were developed with the intent of reducing the side effects associated with MAOIs and CAs. All of the agents in this class inhibit the reuptake of biogenic amines as part of their pharmacologic mechanism of action. In general, the mechanism(s) responsible for overdose-induced seizures for this class of antidepressants remains poorly understood. Duloxetine and reboxetine are not discussed because data are limited regarding overdose with these antidepressant drugs.

Bupropion

Bupropion is an antidepressant that increases the risk of seizures in a dose-related manner. In 1986, it was removed from the US market because of its seizure propensity, especially when patients took high doses.[36] Reintroduced in 1989, it was recommended that total daily doses not exceed 450 mg.[29] Currently, bupropion is indicated for the treatment of depression and used as an adjunct for smoking cessation. It is available in immediate-release (IR), sustained-release (SR), and extended-release (XL) formulations.

The pharmacology of bupropion is not well defined. Bupropion and its active metabolite, hydroxybupropion, inhibit the reuptake of dopamine and, to a lesser degree, norepinephrine and serotonin.[37] Hydroxybupropion may be the causative agent for seizures associated with high therapeutic doses of bupropion or after an overdose. Hydroxybupropion and other metabolites have been detected in much higher concentrations compared with bupropion in patients who have experienced bupropion-induced seizures and in individuals who have died of bupropion overdose.[38,39] However, the precise mechanism for hydroxybupropion-induced seizures remains to be elucidated.

Mirtazapine

Mirtazapine was first introduced for clinical use in 2001 and has a distinctive mechanism of action. It inhibits the reuptake of serotonin; antagonizes H_1 receptors; and antagonizes α_2-adrenergic receptors, which increases neuronal norepinephrine and serotonin concentrations.[40] In addition, mirtazapine blocks some serotonin receptor subtypes including $5\text{-}HT_2$ and $5\text{-}HT_3$.[41] The underlying mechanism for mirtazapine overdose–induced seizures is currently unknown.

Trazodone

The main pharmacologic mechanism of action of trazodone is mediated through antagonism of $5\text{-}HT_{2A}$ receptors and inhibition of serotonin reuptake.[42] It also antagonizes peripheral α_1-adrenergic receptors and has equivocal affinity for H_1 histamine receptors.[24] In rare instances, trazodone can cause hyponatremia through SIADH[43] and this is one reason that may account for seizures after overdose of trazodone.[44]

Venlafaxine

The pathways responsible for seizure activity associated with venlafaxine overdose are likely multiple. This selective norepinephrine/serotonin reuptake inhibitor shares a similar structure and pharmacology to that of tramadol,[45] which has also been reported to cause seizures after overdose.[46] Serotonin toxicity[45] or sodium channel blockade[47] may account for its seizure propensity after intentional ingestion.

EXAMINING THE EVIDENCE FOR ANTIDEPRESSANT OVERDOSE–INDUCED SEIZURES

Before examining the evidence for antidepressant overdose–induced seizures, it is important to recognize the various sources of available clinical data. First and foremost, there are no randomized controlled trials that have evaluated this problem. Much of our knowledge and understanding of antidepressant overdose–induced seizures is based on case reports, case series, observational studies, and retrospective analyses. These methodologies have obvious inherent limitations, and the clinical evidence for antidepressant overdose–induced seizures in many instances may also be hindered by (1) the lack of any control for predisposing risk factors, (2) failure to account for the presence of an underlying seizure disorder, (3) absence of serum drug concentrations, (4) inaccurate reporting of drug doses ingested, or (5) difficulty in determining whether the seizure was caused by the antidepressant or another factor such as a coingestant or a cardiovascular phenomenon that produced a decrease in cerebral perfusion. Nevertheless, these methodologies currently provide the best available evidence with which to evaluate antidepressant overdose–induced seizures in human subjects. **Table 1** provides a quick reference tool that risk stratifies antidepressants for their seizure propensity in overdose.

MAOIs

Reflective of their dwindling use in the clinical arena, human exposures to MAOIs reported to the NPDS in 2009 accounted for only 0.23% (n = 234) of all antidepressant exposures.[2] Seizures after an overdose of a MAOI and with therapeutic use are rare, with few cases reported.[48,49] A subgroup analysis of single-substance overdoses of phenelzine and tranylcypromine reported in a 5-year period found that 2 out of 56 patients who had ingested phenelzine experienced seizure activity, whereas 1 out of 35 patients who had ingested tranylcypromine developed seizure activity.[50] The preponderance of evidence suggests that MAOI overdose–induced seizures typically happen in the setting of polysubstance ingestion or with the development of serotonin syndrome.[51,52] Further supporting this notion is a report that analyzed 106 moclobemide overdose cases.[53] No seizures occurred with the sole ingestion of moclobemide, whereas the concomitant overdose of moclobemide and serotonergic coingestants increased the risk for serotonin syndrome and seizures. Therefore, based on the rarity with which deliberate single-agent ingestions of MAOIs cause seizures, this class of antidepressants should be considered low risk for triggering a seizure after overdose.

CAs

Seizures from CA overdose were reported shortly after the introduction of imipramine in the late 1950s.[54] Since then, a sizeable body of evidence has been published substantiating the propensity for this class of antidepressants to cause seizures in overdose.

Most CA overdose–induced seizures occur within 1 to 2 hours after ingestion and typically are generalized and brief.[55] Status epilepticus with CA poisoning can develop but is unusual. However, seizures from CA poisoning are associated with an increase in mortality,[23] and patients can experience cardiovascular collapse within moments of seizing or while they are seizing.[56] This sudden deterioration is probably caused by enhanced cardiac sodium ion channel blockade that results from the development of a seizure-induced metabolic acidosis.

Several clinical markers have been investigated to predict the risk for developing seizures after CA overdose, including level of consciousness,[57] CA serum concentrations, and QRS duration on the electrocardiogram (ECG).[58] The usefulness of serum CA concentrations after overdose is limited by the difficulty in rapid determination of quantitative CA concentrations and the lack of correlation between life-threatening toxicity and drug concentrations; however, CA serum concentrations greater than 1000 ng/mL are typically linked with significant toxicity.[59] The ECG may aid in predicting which patients are at risk for seizures after CA overdose. For example, one study found that 34% of patients with a QRS duration greater than or equal to 100 milliseconds experienced seizures, whereas no seizures occurred in patients with QRS durations less than 100 milliseconds.[58] Additional studies have shown that a QRS duration greater than 100 milliseconds is associated with serious CA toxicity such as dysrhythmias and seizures.[60,61] However, a normal ECG or QRS duration less than 100 milliseconds cannot be used to exclude the possible development of seizures or other complications after CA overdose.[62,63] A meta-analysis found a pooled sensitivity of

Table 1
Risk stratification for antidepressant overdose–induced seizures[a]

Antidepressant Class Representative Drugs from Each Class	Low Risk <5% Seizure Incidence After Overdose	Intermediate Risk 5%–10% Seizure Incidence After Overdose	High Risk >10% Seizure Incidence After Overdose
MAOIs			
Isocarboxazid[b]	+	−	−
Moclobemide	+	−	−
Phenelzine[b]	+	−	−
Selegiline[b]	+	−	−
Tranylcypromine[b]	+	−	−
CAs			
Tertiary amines			
Amitriptyline	−	+	−
Clomipramine	−	+	−
Doxepin	−	+	−
Imipramine	−	−	+
Trimipramine	−	+	−
Secondary Amines			
Desipramine	−	−	+
Nortriptyline	−	−	+
Protriptyline	−	+	−
Other			
Amoxapine	−	−	+
Maprotiline	−	−	+
SSRIs			
Citalopram[c]	−	+	−
Escitalopram	+	−	−
Fluoxetine	+	−	−
Fluvoxamine	+	−	−
Paroxetine	+	−	−
Sertraline	+	−	−
Atypical Antidepressants			
Bupropion	−	−	+
Duloxetine	Risk unknown	−	−
Mirtazapine	+	−	−
Reboxetine	Risk unknown	−	−
Trazodone	+	−	−
Venlafaxine[d]	−	+	−

[a] Data compiled from multiple sources referenced throughout the article. The table was constructed solely by the authors.

[b] Seizure risk with overdose presumed to be low based on lack of convincing clinical evidence and/or the drug shares a similar structure and/or pharmacologic mechanism to drugs within its class that have been determined to be low risk.

[c] Seizure risk with overdose should be considered high with ingestions exceeding 600 mg.

[d] Seizure risk may be high with large ingestions.

0.69 and specificity of 0.69 for predicting seizures using QRS duration.[64] Comprehensive discussion of prognostic indicators after CA overdose is beyond the scope of this article, and the reader is referred elsewhere for further information.[64]

The incidence of seizures with CA toxicity is varied, ranging from 3% to more than 20%.[65–67] A review that compiled data on 2536 patients from 26 studies of CA overdose reported an overall incidence of 8.4% for CA overdose–induced seizures.[23] An analysis of single-agent suicidal antidepressant ingestions reported to US poison centers from 2000 to 2004 listed the incidence of overdose-induced seizure activity for individual CAs in order of increasing percentage: protriptyline (0%), trimipramine (0%), amitriptyline (3.5%), nortriptyline (4.8%), doxepin (5.2%), clomipramine (6.9%), imipramine (10.5%), and desipramine (14.5%).[50] Other studies with overdose of individual CAs have revealed a high rate of seizures with desipramine (17.9%), imipramine (20.6%), and nortriptyline (22.2%).[65,66] Tabulating the true incidence of seizures for specific CAs is challenging because several of the CAs are infrequently involved in overdose (eg, protriptyline, and trimipramine).[2,50] Based on current knowledge, patients should be stratified as high risk for seizures after toxic ingestions of desipramine, imipramine, and nortriptyline, and intermediate risk for seizures after toxic ingestions of amitriptyline, clomipramine, doxepin, protriptyline, and trimipramine.

Amoxapine

In acute overdose, amoxapine is troublesome. Among 33 patients who overdosed on amoxapine, seizure activity occurred in 36.4% compared with 4.3% in other CA poisonings.[25] This study also showed that the mortality with amoxapine overdose was almost 22 times greater compared with overdose of all other CAs. A study of human exposures to antidepressants reported to the Maryland Poison Control Center in a 2-year period found that 21.7% of patients who had ingested amoxapine alone experienced seizure activity.[65] Moreover, a recent analysis of poison control data found that 29.2% of patients experienced seizure activity after isolated amoxapine ingestions.[50] Because amoxapine overdose has a high likelihood of causing seizures, and because these seizures can be difficult to control,[25] or deteriorate to status epilepticus,[68] this antidepressant should be deemed high risk for causing seizures after overdose.

Maprotiline

There is a significant risk for seizures from maprotiline in acute overdose. A study comparing the relative cardiac and CNS toxicity of amoxapine, maprotiline, and trazodone with older CAs found that 18% of patients developed a seizure after isolated maprotiline overdose.[65] In addition, although only 19 cases of isolated maprotiline ingestions were reported to US poison centers from 2000 to 2004, almost 16% of patients experienced seizure activity.[50] Despite the infrequent use of maprotiline today, it should be labeled high risk for inducing seizure activity after an overdose.

SSRIs

Although this class of antidepressants is believed to be generally safe in overdose, all SSRIs can cause overdose-induced seizures.[30,34] The seizure risk from escitalopram, fluoxetine, fluvoxamine, paroxetine, and sertraline overdose is low. A prospective multicenter study that analyzed 87 cases of isolated fluoxetine ingestion reported no seizures.[69] In a cohort study of 233 first admissions of deliberate self-poisoning with a single SSRI, seizures occurred in only 1.3% of patients.[45] A retrospective cohort study that compared the clinical features of deliberate self-poisoning with venlafaxine and SSRIs reported a seizure rate of 2.3% after SSRI overdose.[70] A review of SSRI poisoning admissions to an Australian toxicology unit reported a seizure incidence of 2% for citalopram, 1% for fluoxetine, 4% for fluvoxamine, 2% for paroxetine, and 2% for sertraline.[30]

Several retrospective reviews evaluating monointoxication with either citalopram or escitalopram have revealed that citalopram has a greater tendency for causing seizures after overdose. First, Ho and colleagues[71] found that seizures occurred in 7.5% of patients who ingested citalopram (median dose 536 mg) alone compared with 3% of patients who ingested escitalopram (median dose 222 mg) alone. Second, Hayes and colleagues[35] evaluated single-substance acute overdoses with citalopram and escitalopram; seizures were described more commonly with citalopram (8%) than with escitalopram (0.2%). Third, isolated citalopram and escitalopram overdoses reported to several European poison centers from 1997 to 2006 were retrospectively analyzed; seizures occurred in 13.6% of cases after citalopram overdose compared with 1.6% after escitalopram overdose.[34] When seizures occur after citalopram overdose, they are typically generalized, self-limited, or terminate with benzodiazepines, and develop within 1 to 13 hours after ingestion.[72]

The risk of citalopram overdose–induced seizures escalates in a dose-related fashion. Waring and colleagues[72] found that, in the absence of coingestants, the minimum dose of citalopram associated with seizures was 400 mg. Hayes and colleagues[35] reported a 3% incidence of seizures in patients ingesting less than 600 mg citalopram, 11.6% seizure incidence for ingestions between 600 and 1900 mg, and 75% incidence of seizures for ingestions greater than 1900 mg. A study by Yilmaz and colleagues[34] showed seizures in 11% of cases at doses of 400 to 800 mg citalopram; 27% of cases at doses of 802 to 1200 mg; 41% of cases at doses of 1202 to 1600 mg; and 52% of cases at doses greater than 1600 mg. Clinical evidence for citalopram overdose–induced seizures continues to mount. Although it is difficult to determine an exact dose at which seizures will occur with citalopram overdose, current data suggest that this antidepressant should be categorized as intermediate risk with ingestions between 400 and 600 mg, and high risk when doses exceed 600 mg.

ATYPICAL ANTIDEPRESSANTS
Bupropion

Several studies have shown that the IR, SR, and XL formulations of bupropion have a high incidence of seizures in overdose.[73–75] Seizure activity occurred in 21% of patients with overdose involving the IR formulation,[73] 11% of patients who primarily overdosed on the SR formulation,[74] and 32% of patients who overdosed on the XL formulation.[75] Seizures induced by overdose of bupropion are problematic because they can be multiple[50] and can progress to status epilepticus.[5] As an example, analysis of US poison control data from 2000 to 2004 revealed 7631 cases of solitary bupropion ingestions; 801 cases involved a single seizure, 450 cases involved multiple seizures, and 61 cases involved status epilepticus.[50] Furthermore, Starr and colleagues[75] reported that almost one-half of the patients in their observational study of bupropion XL overdoses had experienced more than 1 seizure.

Another problem with bupropion overdose–induced seizures is the delayed onset with which they can occur. Seizure activity has been reported to occur up to 8 hours (mean, 3.7 hours),[73] 14 hours (mean, 4.3 hours),[74] and 24 hours (mean, 7.3 hours)[75] after overdose on the IR, SR, and XL preparations, respectively. Even though patients who develop a bupropion overdose–induced seizure are more likely to have agitation or tremor on physical examination before seizing, these seizures can develop in patients lacking any signs or symptoms of CNS toxicity.[75] Based on the high incidence of seizures after overdose of bupropion, and because these seizures can be multiple or delayed in their onset, this drug should be labeled as high risk after overdose.

Mirtazapine

Not much is known about mirtazapine overdose and data continue to accumulate. A retrospective chart review of mirtazapine ingestions reported to a US poison center in 2004 identified 33 intentional and isolated mirtazapine ingestions; no seizures were reported to have occurred.[41] Mirtazapine accounted for 3.1% (n = 2599) of single-agent suicidal antidepressant ingestions reported to US poison centers from 2000 to 2004 and a single seizure occurred in 5 cases.[50] A retrospective analysis reported no seizure activity with 117 cases of mirtazapine overdose admitted to a Scottish toxicology unit during a 5-year period.[40] However, the investigators of the same study postulated that, given the study size, a power of 87% to detect a 3% risk of seizures, and assuming a background frequency of 0.1%, that the true risk of seizures with mirtazapine overdose could be as high as 2.6%. Existing evidence supports that this antidepressant is low risk for overdose-induced seizures.

Trazodone

With the exception of CNS depression and mild hypotension, the effects of trazodone when ingested as a single agent in deliberate self-poisonings are not severe.[76] Seizures have been reported after trazodone overdose but are uncommon.[77] Between the years 2000 and 2004, trazodone accounted for 15.1% (n = 12,538) of single-agent suicidal antidepressant ingestions reported to US poison centers, and a single seizure occurred in 13 cases.[50] Because seizures have been shown to occur only sporadically after the intentional ingestion of trazodone as a sole agent, this atypical antidepressant should be categorized as low risk for overdose-induced seizures.

Venlafaxine

Venlafaxine was previously considered to have low toxicity with overdose compared with MAOIs and CAs.[17] However, newer evidence from a comparison of fatality indices suggests that venlafaxine is more toxic than SSRIs and at least as toxic as clomipramine and nortriptyline.[78] Venlafaxine has shown a greater proclivity toward seizures with overdose compared with drugs within some of the other antidepressant classes. In a 2003 prospective cohort study, seizures occurred in approximately 14% of venlafaxine overdoses and were more frequent than SSRI and tricyclic antidepressant overdose–induced seizures.[45] All of the patients who had experienced a venlafaxine overdose–induced seizure had ingested 900 mg or more. In a comparative analysis performed by White and colleagues,[50] venlafaxine caused seizure activity in 220 out of 5510 patients (~4%) who had ingested it in a suicidal overdose; 11 of the patients were reported to have experienced status epilepticus. Recently, a retrospective cohort study assessed 36 patients with venlafaxine self-poisoning and 44 randomly selected patients with SSRI self-poisoning; seizures were recorded in 8.3% of the venlafaxine cases compared with 2.3% of the SSRI cases.[70] Because there is an evolving body of evidence that continues to reveal the proconvulsant effects of venlafaxine with overdose, it should be ranked as intermediate risk for overdose-induced seizures; however, large ingestions may increase this risk.

TREATMENT CONSIDERATIONS

Evaluating and treating a patient who has overdosed on an antidepressant can pose several challenges to the clinician.

1. Patients may present with altered mental status, significantly limiting the ability to take an adequate history.
2. The patient may have ingested other substances contributing to their clinical presentation.
3. Some antidepressants, such as bupropion and citalopram, can cause delayed-onset seizures.
4. Antidepressant overdose–induced seizures can deteriorate to status epilepticus.
5. In addition to causing neurotoxicity, several antidepressants can result in life-threatening cardiotoxicity that requires prompt antidotal therapy.

After assessing the patient's airway and vital signs, a focused history should be obtained and a physical examination performed. The exposure history can be supported by findings on the physical examination such as agitation, CNS depression, diaphoresis, mydriasis, or tachycardia. The patient may have a specific toxidrome after ingestion of an antidepressant (eg, anticholinergic from CA overdose, serotonin syndrome from SSRI overdose, or sympathomimetic from MAOI or venlafaxine overdose). Intravenous access should be established, and the patient placed on a cardiac monitor and under seizure precautions. Although the benefits of gastrointestinal decontamination are controversial,[79] activated charcoal at a dose of 1 g/kg should be considered when an ingestion of an antidepressant is potentially life-threatening, or an SR formulation was ingested. To decrease the likelihood of aspiration, awake patients should be able to protect their airway or, if a patient is intubated, the airway should be secured with a cuffed endotracheal tube before administration of activated charcoal.

Because many poisoned patients are unable or unwilling to provide a reliable history, laboratory evaluation is crucial. Rapid determination of blood glucose should be performed for all patients with altered mental status or those who are actively seizing. Diagnostic tests, such as a comprehensive metabolic panel and ECG, provide invaluable information regarding end-organ toxicity and insight into potential deterioration in a patient's condition. A quantitative test for common coingestants, for instance acetaminophen or aspirin, may be warranted, whereas quantitative testing of specific antidepressants is not recommended. The routine use of serum and urine drug screens in the acute overdose patient is infrequently beneficial.

Risk factors for seizures should be identified and include history of seizures, head trauma, polypharmacy, CNS lesions, and concomitant substance abuse or withdrawal.[27] **Table 1** can be used to help determine the risk of seizures after overdose of various antidepressants. If the patient is actively seizing, benzodiazepines such as diazepam, lorazepam, or midazolam are considered first-line therapy. Second-line therapy includes phenobarbital. If large doses of these agents are used, or if the patient develops refractory seizures, then intubation may be necessary for airway protection and ventilation. If neuromuscular blockade is necessary to facilitate intubation, then a nondepolarizing agent with a short duration of action, like rocuronium, should be used.[80] The use of long-acting paralytics should be avoided; however, if a drug such as pancuronium has to be used, then bedside electroencephalographic monitoring should be instituted.

If seizures are refractory to benzodiazepine and barbiturate therapy, propofol has been used successfully used to treat antidepressant overdose-induced seizures.[68]

Patients who develop refractory seizures from ingestions of a hydrazine derivate, or when the ingestion is unknown, should be treated with pyridoxine. Phenytoin, although second-line therapy for most seizures, is usually not effective for the treatment of drug-induced seizures or CA overdose–induced seizures.[6,81] Patients who are seizing from an antidepressant that causes cardiac sodium channel blockade should be treated simultaneously with 1 to 2 mEq/kg of sodium bicarbonate given as an intravenous bolus in addition to conventional therapy and repeated as needed until a blood pH of 7.55 is attained[82,83]; sodium bicarbonate is effective for treating drug-induced cardiac sodium channel blockade.[84] In addition, lipid emulsion, a novel therapy believed to work by pulling lipid-soluble drugs out of tissues, has been used to successfully restore circulation in a patient who experienced seizure activity and cardiovascular collapse after overdose of bupropion and lamotrigine.[85]

The process of determining disposition after an antidepressant overdose is not always straightforward. Any patient who has overdosed on an antidepressant and is displaying signs or symptoms of toxicity should be admitted for further evaluation and treatment. In many instances, patients can be observed for a period of 4 to 6 hours after ingestion. If they remain without signs or symptoms of toxicity, a decision on disposition can be rendered; the patient may require psychiatric evaluation or can be discharged home. Patients who have ingested CAs and who are asymptomatic on presentation, receive activated charcoal, remain asymptomatic for a minimum of 6 hours in the treating facility without any treatment intervention, and have normal ECGs can receive disposition as deemed appropriate.[86] Some exceptions that necessitate prolonged monitoring include ingestion of (1) sustained-release formulations, (2) drugs that can cause delayed-onset seizures (eg, bupropion or citalopram), or (3) antidepressants that can cause cardiotoxicity, such as bupropion,[85] citalopram and escitalopram,[35] or venlafaxine.[45]

SUMMARY

Deliberate self-ingestion of antidepressants is a problem commonly encountered in emergency departments throughout the United States. Because seizures are a serious complication of antidepressant overdose, clinicians should recognize the risk associated with overdose of various antidepressants. Understanding the seizure potential of antidepressants in overdose can help to determine the need for inpatient monitoring and assist in treatment decisions for clinicians.

REFERENCES

1. Olfson M, Marcus SC. National patterns in antidepressant medication treatment. Arch Gen Psychiatry 2009;66:848–56.
2. Bronstein AC, Spyker DA, Cantilena LR Jr, et al. 2009 annual report of the American Association of Poison Control Centers' National Poison Data System (NPDS): 27th Annual Report. Clin Toxicol 2010;48:979–1178.
3. Beuhler MC, Spiller HA, Sasser HC. The outcome of unintentional pediatric bupropion ingestions: a NPDS database review. J Med Toxicol 2010;6:4–8.
4. Pisani F, Oteri G, Costa C, et al. Effects of psychotropic drugs on seizure threshold. Drug Saf 2002;25:91–110.
5. Thundiyil JG, Kearney TE, Olson KR. Evolving epidemiology of drug-induced seizures reported to a poison control center system. J Med Toxicol 2007;3:15–9.
6. Wills B, Erickson T. Chemically induced seizures. Clin Lab Med 2006;26:185–209.
7. Clark M, Post RM. Carbamazepine, but not caffeine, is highly selective for adenosine A_1 binding sites. Eur J Pharmacol 1989;164:399–401.

8. Malatynska E, Knapp RJ, Ikeda M, et al. Antidepressants and seizure-interactions at the GABA-receptor chloride-ionophore complex. Life Sci 1988;43:303–7.

9. Yokoyama H, Iinuma K. Histamine and seizures: implications for the treatment of epilepsy. CNS Drugs 1996;5:321–30.

10. Tuovinen K. Organophosphate-induced convulsions and prevention of neuro-pathological damages. Toxicology 2004;196:31–9.

11. Teitelbaum JS, Zatorre RJ, Carpenter S, et al. Neurologic sequelae of domoic acid intoxication due to the ingestion of contaminated mussels. N Engl J Med 1990;322:1781–7.

12. DeToledo JC. Lidocaine and seizures. Ther Drug Monit 2000;22:320–2.

13. Jobe PC, Browning RA. The serotonergic and noradrenergic effects of antide-pressant drugs are anticonvulsant, not proconvulsant. Epilepsy Behav 2005;7:602–19.

14. Dailey JW, Naritoku DK. Antidepressants and seizures: clinical anecdotes over-shadow neuroscience. Biochem Pharmacol 1996;52:1323–9.

15. Krishnan KR. Revisiting monoamine oxidase inhibitors. J Clin Psychiatry 2007;68(Suppl 8):35–41.

16. Bonnet U. Moclobemide: evolution, pharmacodynamic, and pharmacokinetic properties. CNS Drug Rev 2002;8:283–308.

17. Richelson E. Pharmacology of antidepressants. Mayo Clin Proc 2001;76:511–27.

18. Frieling H, Bleich S. Tranylcypromine: new perspectives on an "old" drug. Eur Arch Psychiatry Clin Neurosci 2006;256:268–73.

19. Bonnet U. Moclobemide: therapeutic use and clinical studies. CNS Drug Rev 2003;9:97–140.

20. Judge BS. Differentiating the causes of metabolic acidosis in the poisoned patient. Clin Lab Med 2006;26:31–48.

21. Squires RF, Saederup H. Antidepressants and metabolites that block GABA$_A$ receptors coupled to ^{35}S-t-butylbicyclophosphorothionate binding sites in rat brain. Brain Res 1988;441:15–22.

22. Shioda K, Nisijima K, Yoshino T, et al. Extracellular serotonin, dopamine and glutamate levels are elevated in the hypothalamus in a serotonin syndrome animal model induced by tranylcypromine and fluoxetine. Prog Neuropsycho-pharmacol Biol Psychiatry 2004;28:633–40.

23. Frommer DA, Kulig KW, Marx JA, et al. Tricyclic antidepressant overdose. JAMA 1987;257:521–6.

24. Rudorfer MV, Manji HK, Potter WZ. Comparative tolerability profiles of the newer versus older antidepressants. Drug Saf 1994;10:18–46.

25. Litovitz TL, Troutman WG. Amoxapine overdose: seizures and fatalities. JAMA 1983;250:1069–71.

26. Kumlien E, Lundberg PO. Seizure risk associated with neuroactive drugs: Data from the WHO adverse drug reactions database. Seizure 2010;19:69–73.

27. Skowron DM, Stimmel GL. Antidepressants and the risk of seizures. Pharmaco-therapy 1992;12:18–22.

28. Jabbari B, Bryan GE, March EE, et al. Incidence of seizures with tricyclic and tet-racyclic antidepressants. Arch Neurol 1985;42:480–1.

29. Lee KC, Finley PR, Alldredge BK. Risk of seizures associated with psychotropic medications: emphasis on new drugs and new findings. Expert Opin Drug Saf 2003;2:233–47.

30. Isbister GK, Bowe SJ, Dawson A, et al. Relative toxicity of selective serotonin re-uptake inhibitors (SSRIs) in overdose. J Toxicol Clin Toxicol 2004;42:277–85.

31. Suchard JR. Fluoxetine overdose-induced seizure. West J Emerg Med 2008;9:154–6.

32. Kirchner V, Silver LE, Kelly CA. Selective serotonin reuptake inhibitors and hypo-natraemia: review and proposed mechanisms in the elderly. J Psychopharmacol 1998;12:396–400.

33. Corrington KA, Gatlin CC, Fields KB. A case of SSRI-induced hyponatremia. J Am Board Fam Pract 2002;15:63–5.

34. Yilmaz Z, Ceschi A, Rauber-Lüthy C, et al. Escitalopram causes fewer seizures in human overdose than citalopram. Clin Toxicol 2010;48:207–12.

35. Hayes BD, Klein-Schwartz W, Clark RF, et al. Comparison of toxicity of acute over-doses with citalopram and escitalopram. J Emerg Med 2010;39:44–8.

36. Alldredge BK. Seizure risk associated with psychotropic drugs: clinical and phar-macokinetic considerations. Neurology 1999;53(Suppl 2):S68–75.

37. Ascher JA, Cole JO, Colin JN, et al. Bupropion: a review of its mechanism of anti-depressant activity. J Clin Psychiatry 1995;56:395–401.

38. Friel PN, Logan BK, Fligner CL. Three fatal drug overdoses involving bupropion. J Anal Toxicol 1993;17:436–8.

39. Davidson J. Seizures and bupropion: a review. J Clin Psychiatry 1989;50: 256–61.

40. Waring WS, Good AM, Bateman DN. Lack of significant toxicity after mirtazapine overdose: a five-year review of cases admitted to a regional toxicology unit. Clin Toxicol 2007;45:45–50.

41. LoVecchio F, Riley B, Pizon A, et al. Outcomes after isolated mirtazapine (Remeron) supratherapeutic ingestions. J Emerg Med 2008;34:77–8.

42. Montgomery SA. Antidepressants and seizures: emphasis on newer agents and clinical implications. Int J Clin Pract 2005;59:1435–40.

43. Spigset O, Hedenmalm K. Hyponatraemia and the syndrome of inappropriate antidiuretic hormone secretion (SIADH) induced by psychotropic drugs. Drug Saf 1995;12:209–25.

44. Vanpee D, Laloyaux P, Gillet JB. Seizure and hyponatremia after overdose of tra-zodone. Am J Emerg Med 1999;17:430–1.

45. Whyte IM, Dawson AH, Buckley NA. Relative toxicity of venlafaxine and selective serotonin reuptake inhibitors in overdose compared to tricyclic antidepressants. QJM 2003;96:369–74.

46. Tobias J. Seizure after overdose of tramadol. South Med J 1997;90:826–7.

47. Khalifa M, Daleau P, Turgeon J. Mechanism of sodium channel block by venlafax-ine in guinea pig ventricular myocytes. J Pharmacol Exp Ther 1999;291:280–4.

48. Bhugra DK, Kaye N. Phenelizine induced grand mal seizure. Br J Clin Pract 1986; 40:173–4.

49. Albareda M, Udina C, Escartín A, et al. Seizures in a diabetic patient on mono-amine oxidase inhibitors. Am J Emerg Med 1999;17:107–8.

50. White NC, Litovitz T, Clancy C. Suicidal antidepressant overdoses: a comparative analysis by antidepressant type. J Med Toxicol 2008;4:238–50.

51. Vouri E, Henry JA, Ojanperä I, et al. Death following ingestion of MDMA (ecstasy) and moclobemide. Addiction 2003;98:365–8.

52. Singer PP, Jones GR. An uncommon fatality due to moclobemide. J Anal Toxicol 1997;21:518–20.

53. Isbister GK, Hackett LP, Dawson AH, et al. Moclobemide poisoning: toxicoki-netics and occurrence of serotonin toxicity. Br J Clin Pharmacol 2003;56:441–50.

54. Zaccara G, Muscas GC, Messori A. Clinical features, pathogenesis and manage-ment of drug-induced seizures. Drug Saf 1990;5:109–51.

55. Ellison DW, Pentel PR. Clinical features and consequences of seizures due to cyclic antidepressant overdose. Am J Emerg Med 1989;7:5–10.

56. Taboulet P, Michard R, Muszynski J, et al. Cardiovascular repercussions of seizures during cyclic antidepressant poisoning. J Toxicol Clin Toxicol 1995;33: 205–11.
57. Hultén BÅ, Adams R, Askenasi R, et al. Predicting severity of tricyclic antidepressant overdose. J Toxicol Clin Toxicol 1992;30:161–70.
58. Boehnert MT, Lovejoy FH Jr. Value of the QRS duration versus the serum drug level in predicting seizures and ventricular arrhythmias after an acute overdose of tricyclic antidepressants. N Engl J Med 1985;313:474–9.
59. Lavoie FW, Gansert GG, Weiss RE. Value of initial ECG findings and plasma drug levels in cyclic antidepressant overdose. Ann Emerg Med 1990;19:696–700.
60. Caravati EM, Bossart PJ. Demographic and electrocardiographic factors associated with severe tricyclic antidepressant toxicity. J Toxicol Clin Toxicol 1991;29: 31–43.
61. Leibelt EL, Francis PD, Woolf AD. ECG lead aVR versus QRS interval in predicting seizures and arrhythmias in acute tricyclic antidepressant toxicity. Ann Emerg Med 1995;26:195–201.
62. Buckley NA, Dawson AH. Greater toxicity in overdose of dothiepin than of other tricyclic antidepressants. Lancet 1994;343:159–62.
63. Foulke GE, Albertson TE. QRS interval in tricyclic antidepressant overdosage: inaccuracy as a toxicity indicator in emergency settings. Ann Emerg Med 1987;16: 160–3.
64. Bailey B, Buckley NA, Amre DK. A meta-analysis of prognostic indicators to predict seizures, arrhythmias, or death after tricyclic antidepressant overdose. J Toxicol Clin Toxicol 2004;42:877–88.
65. Wedin GP, Oderda GM, Klein-Schwartz W. Relative toxicity of cyclic antidepressants. Ann Emerg Med 1986;15:797–804.
66. Crome P, Newman B. The problem of tricyclic antidepressant poisoning. Postgrad Med J 1979;55:528–32.
67. Strøm J, Madsen PS, Nielsen NN, et al. Acute self-poisoning with tricyclic antidepressants in 295 consecutive patients treated in an ICU. Acta Anaesthesiol Scand 1984;28:666–70.
68. Merigian KS, Browning RG, Leeper KV. Successful treatment of amoxapine-induced refractory status epilepticus with propofol (Diprivan). Acad Emerg Med 1995;2:128–33.
69. Borys DJ, Setzer SC, Ling LJ, et al. Acute fluoxetine overdose: a report of 234 cases. Am J Emerg Med 1992;10:115–20.
70. Chan AN, Gunja N, Ryan CJ. A comparison of venlafaxine and SSRIs in deliberate self-poisoning. J Med Toxicol 2010;6:116–21.
71. Ho R, Norman RF, van Veen MM, et al. A 3-year review of citalopram and escitalopram ingestions [abstract]. J Toxicol Clin Toxicol 2004;42:746.
72. Waring WS, Gray JA, Graham A. Predictive factors for generalized seizures after deliberate citalopram overdose. Br J Clin Pharmacol 2008;66:861–5.
73. Spiller HA, Ramoska EA, Sheen SR, et al. Bupropion overdose: a 3-year multicenter retrospective analysis. Am J Emerg Med 1994;12:43–5.
74. Shepherd G, Velez LI, Keyes DC. Intentional bupropion overdoses. J Emerg Med 2004;27:147–51.
75. Starr P, Klein-Schwartz W, Spiller H, et al. Incidence and onset of delayed seizures after overdoses of extended-release bupropion. Am J Emerg Med 2009;27:911–5.
76. Sarko J. Antidepressants, old and new: a review of their adverse effects and toxicity in overdose. Emerg Med Clin North Am 2000;18:637–54.

77. Gamble DE. Trazodone overdose: four years of experience from voluntary reports. J Clin Psychiatry 1986;47:544–6.
78. Buckley NA, McManus PR. Fatal toxicity of serotoninergic and other antidepressant drugs: analysis of United Kingdom mortality data. BMJ 2002;325:1332–3.
79. Heard K. The changing indications of gastrointestinal decontamination. Clin Lab Med 2006;26:1–12.
80. Marik PE, Varon J. The management of status epilepticus. Chest 2004;126: 582–91.
81. Pimentel L, Trommer L. Cyclic antidepressant overdoses: a review. Emerg Med Clin North Am 1994;12:533–47.
82. Smilkstein MJ. Reviewing cyclic antidepressant cardiotoxicity: wheat and chaff. J Emerg Med 1990;8:645–8.
83. Pentel PR, Benowitz NL. Tricyclic antidepressant poisoning. Management of arrhythmias. Med Toxicol 1986;1:101–21.
84. Hoffman JR, Votey SR, Bayer M, et al. Effect of hypertonic sodium bicarbonate in the treatment of moderate-to-severe cyclic antidepressant overdose. Am J Emerg Med 1993;11:336–41.
85. Sirianni AJ, Osterhoudt KC, Calello DP, et al. Use of lipid emulsion in the resuscitation of a patient with prolonged cardiovascular collapse after overdose of bupropion and lamotrigine. Ann Emerg Med 2008;51:412–5.
86. Banahan BF Jr, Schelkun PH. Tricyclic antidepressant overdose: conservative management in a community hospital with cost-saving implications. J Emerg Med 1990;8:451–4.

A Brief Review of Cognitive Assessment in Neurotoxicology

Dong (Dan) Y. Han, PsyD[a],*, James B. Hoelzle, PhD[b],
Brandon C. Dennis, PsyD[a], Michael Hoffmann, MD[c]

KEYWORDS

• Cognitive testing • Cognitive assessment • Neurotoxicology
• Neurotoxicity

Among commercial and industrial chemicals, cosmetics, food additives, pesticides, and medicinal drugs, there are more than 50,000 substances distributed. Of these, approximately 600 have standards set by Occupational Safety and Health Administration (OSHA) and approximately 200 have been regulated for neurotoxic effects.[1–3] The major categories of neurotoxic insults to the brain include: (1) heavy metals, (2) industrial toxins and solvents, (3) venom bites, stings, and plant poisons, (4) bacterial toxins, (5) addictive drugs such as opiates, and synthetic analgesics, (6) sedative hypnotic drugs, (7) antidepressants and antipsychotic drugs, (8) psychoactive drugs and stimulants, and (9) antineoplastic and immunosuppressive drugs.[3] Any of these may pose neurotoxic effects that can incur cognitive impairment, especially with prolonged exposure. Accordingly, a systematic method of tracking cognitive changes is pertinent to clinical practice. As bedside neurologic examinations may be insufficient in tracking more subtle cognitive sequelae of neurotoxic exposure, extended neurocognitive testing is proposed to better understand individual clinical presentation.

CLINICAL MANIFESTATIONS OF NEUROTOXICITY

There are two broad categories of neurotoxicity: neuropsychological impairments and elementary neurologic impairments.[3] Neuropsychological impairments may include declines in attention/concentration, memory (especially short-term memory),

[a] Department of Neurology, University of Kentucky College of Medicine, 740 South Limestone Street, Suite L445, Lexington, KY 40536-0284, USA
[b] Department of Psychology, Marquette University, PO Box 1881, Milwaukee, WI 53201-1881, USA
[c] Department of Neurology, James A. Haley Veteran's Hospital, 13000 Bruce Down's Boulevard, Tampa, FL 33612, USA
* Corresponding author. Department of Neurology, University of Kentucky College of Medicine, 740 South Limestone Street, Suite L445, Lexington, KY 40536-0284.
E-mail address: d.han@uky.edu

Neurol Clin 29 (2011) 581–590
doi:10.1016/j.ncl.2011.05.008
0733-8619/11/$ – see front matter © 2011 Elsevier Inc. All rights reserved.

executive functioning, processing speed, language, visuospatial skills, depression, and anxiety. Elementary neurologic presentations may include toxic neuropathies, myopathies, tremor, parkinsonism, myoclonus, dystonia, ballismus, and tics, to name a few.[3]

Given the myriad of possible symptom presentations, a formal neuropsychological test should be viewed as an extension of the neurologic examination. These tests are particularly useful in assessing for particular toxin-derived syndromes. Most patients with neurotoxicity present with impairments in the cognitive domains of attention, executive functioning, and memory.[3] However, it has been documented that other clinical syndromes may be correlated with toxic exposure, further complicating the cognitive sequelae beyond that of a mechanism exclusive to acute neurotoxicity.

As an example, there is evidence for a relationship between solvent exposure and neurodegenerative disease such as Alzheimer disease (AD). Years of solvent exposure ($\geq$2000 workplace exposure hours) is correlated with an increased risk of AD.[4] In a community-based study of solvent (benzene, toluene, phenols, alcohols, and ketones) exposure and AD, an odds ratio of 2.3 (95% confidence interval [CI]: 1.1–4.7) was identified. With men, the odds ratio was 6.0 (95% CI: 2.1–17.2).[3,5]

Additional clinical manifestations of neurotoxicity include serotonin syndrome and toxin-induced posterior reversible encephalopathy syndrome (PRES). Serotonin syndrome is characterized by the following: (1) neuromuscular excitation, (2) autonomic stimulation, and (3) altered cognition (confusion, anxiety, obtundation, and coma). The syndrome has been described as being caused by selective serotonin reuptake inhibitors, monoamine oxidase inhibitors, and atypical antipsychotic agents.[3] The pathophysiology of serotonin syndrome is a hyperserotonergic state of the central and the peripheral nervous systems.[6] PRES is characterized by symptoms such as cortical blindness, headaches, seizures, and possible simultanagnosia and Balint syndrome. Etiologic factors include exposure to cyclosporin, tacrolimus, FK 506, methotrexate, interferon, cisplatin, cytarabine, L-asparaginase, intravenous immunoglobulin, erythropoietin, and granulocyte-colony stimulating factor. As this is a reversible syndrome, with proper management patients can return to their baseline functioning level fairly quickly.[3]

It has also been documented that there is an increased risk of attention deficit/hyperactivity disorder (ADHD) associated with early exposure to lead, pesticides, and polychlorinated biphenyls (PCBs). Data suggest that lead may reduce attention and response inhibition, whereas PCBs impair response inhibition more than attention.[7,8] Again, given all these different disease associations and clinical manifestations of neurotoxic exposure, a comprehensive approach to cognitive assessment is essential for high-quality clinical management.

COGNITIVE ASSESSMENT FOR PATIENTS WITH NEUROTOXICOLOGIC SYNDROME

As noted, most patients with neurotoxicity present with impairments in attention, executive functioning, and memory.[3] However, posttoxic exposure cognitive impairment is not necessarily limited to these domains. To provide a thorough assessment of posttoxic exposure, neurologic examination and extended metric assessment should cover the following: (1) level of consciousness, (2) orientation, (3) attention/concentration, (4) aphasias, dysarthrias, (5) frontal network syndromes, (6) amnesias, (7) alexias, (8) anosognosias and neglect syndromes, (9) visuospatial deficit, (10) right/left orientation, (11) naming, (12) apraxias, appendicular and axial, (13) acalculias, (14) agraphias, (15) alexias, (16) agnosias, (17) complex visual syndromes: simultanagnosia, prosopagnosia, (18) achromatopsias, and (19) illusions, and hallucinations, with inquiry into content-specific delusions.[3]

The advantages of metric cognitive evaluation over bedside cognitive assessment include standardized administration and scoring guidelines, documented reliability and validity, tracking ability through serial testing, and availability of normative values.[3] This approach is also endorsed by the guidelines issued by the American Academy of Neurology.[9]

Regarding the use of neuropsychological/psychometric tests, it is imperative to consider a patient's level of engagement when interpreting performance. Because clinicians are notoriously poor at determining whether sufficient motivation is present during evaluations, there have been successful efforts to develop techniques to more formally evaluate effort.[10,11] There is compelling evidence that this issue might be especially important in the context of suspected chronic toxic encephalopathy.[12] This issue also becomes more pertinent should there be any pending medicolegal/litigation involvement.

COGNITIVE ASSESSMENT TOOLS COMMONLY EMPLOYED IN NEUROPSYCHOLOGY
Measures of Attention/Concentration

Trail-making test
The trail-making test (TMT) was originally developed as part of the Army Individual Test Battery (1944). It is a relatively brief test of visual scanning and sustained attention that consists of two trials. The first trial requires examinees to rapidly draw lines connecting numbers in order; the second requires an individual to alternate drawing lines connecting numbers and letters (eg, 1-A-2-B, and so forth). The latter trial is assumed to be a more cognitively demanding task because set shifting is required. Total time necessary to complete each trial is interpreted as an indication of attentional ability. Errors are not interpreted per se, though during administration examinees are required to correct errors as they occur, so that committing numerous errors will affect overall performance. Researchers have considered the ratio of performance across trials in an attempt to develop a more sensitive index of cognitive flexibility that controls for intrasubject variability.[13]

Stroop test
The Stroop test consists of 3 relatively brief trials that require examinees to rapidly (1) read the names of colors, (2) name colors, and (3) name the color of a printed incongruent color word (eg, the word blue printed in red ink).[14] The latter trial is referred to as the interference trial because it requires one to override an overlearned reading response. Performance on the interference trial is associated with activation of the anterior cingulate and left frontal cortex.[15] Clinicians should be aware that slightly different versions of the Stroop test are available and have different administration procedures. In general, similar classification of impairment occurs across forms. Also, it is imperative that examinees be able to differentiate between test stimuli colors for valid administration.

Visual Search and Attention Test
The Visual Search and Attention Test (VSAT) is primarily an attention test that aims to measure sustained attention, which is an important component of information processing.[16] The VSAT utilizes visual cancellation tasks to measure sustained attention, including a searching task for letters, symbols, and colors.[3]

Measures of Executive Functioning

Wisconsin Card-Sorting Test
The Wisconsin Card-Sorting Test (WCST) is a well-regarded test of frontal function or executive (metacognitive) function that is scored according to several different criteria.[17] Given that the task requires an examinee to sort test stimuli according to

color, similar to the Stroop test, it is essential to determine whether different colors can be perceived prior to administration. In a broad sense, the test evaluates abstraction and ability to shift problem-solving strategies in the context of changing contingencies. A computer-administrated or examiner-administered 128 (or 64) card test is employed, and examples of scoring variables include, but are not limited to: (1) Trials to Complete First Category, (2) Categories Completed, (3) Failure to Maintain Set, (4) % Conceptual Level Responses, (5) Learning to Learn, (6) Total Errors, (7) Perseverative Errors, and (8) Nonperseverative Errors. Clinicians should be aware that there are several redundancies between WCST scoring variables and, as a result, scores are highly correlated with one another. "Categories Completed" and number of "Perservative Errors" are most often interpreted as reflecting executive control. There is evidence that the latter might be slightly more sensitive as a metric of executive dysfunction.[18] Also, there is compelling empirical evidence suggesting that an excessive number of failures to maintain set errors indicates incomplete effort.[19]

Delis-Kaplan Executive Function Systems Test

The Delis-Kaplan Executive Function Systems (D-KEFS) test was designed to evaluate mild forms of executive dysfunction.[20] The test comprises 9 subtests, many of which are similar to traditional neuropsychological measures such as the Stroop test or TMT. The advantage of administering a D-KEFS test over a traditional measure of attention or executive function is that D-KEFS tasks were developed to increase processing demands. For example, whereas the traditional TMT included 2 trials (Numbers; Number-Letter), the D-KEFS TMT consists of 5 trials (Scanning; Numbers; Letters; Number-Letter; Direct Processing Speed). Interpretation of these trials may facilitate greater understanding as to why a more complex task is not efficiently completed. Theoretically, changes made to traditional neuropsychological tests should increase sensitivity to mild brain dysfunction. An additional strength of the D-KEFS test is that clinicians can compare an individual's level of performance with that of a large normative sample demographically consistent with the 2000 census. Although it is more time intensive than traditional measures, clinicians can use the D-KEFS test in a flexible manner and are free to administer any or all of the following tests to evaluate executive functioning: (1) trail-making test, (2) verbal fluency test, (3) design fluency test, (4) color-word interference test, (5) sorting test, (6) twenty-questions test, (7) word-context test, (8) tower test, and (9) proverb test. It should be noted that select D-KEFS tests are not revised versions of frequently used tests (eg, twenty-questions test or word-context test), and relatively little is known about neurologic correlates.

Tower tests

Tower tests require a subject to determine and complete a series of steps to rearrange rings or balls so that they are consistent with a goal. Various versions of the test have been developed. For example, a noncomprehensive list of similar tasks includes the Tower of London,[21] Tower of Hanoi,[22] and the D-KEFS[20] Tower Test. Scoring is generally determined based on number of total moves required and completion time. Sequencing errors that occur while completing the task are often interpreted. It is important to recognize that there are subtle differences between versions of tower tests. Discrepant administration procedures and task requirements may result in evaluation of different cognitive abilities.[23] In general, successful completion of the test requires planning ability, working memory, response inhibition, and visual memory.[24] Imaging studies have documented heightened activation of the prefrontal cortex during task completion.[25] Tower tests have also been shown to be sensitive to frontal lobe dysfunction due to both unilateral and bilateral disease.

Measures of Memory

List-learning tests

Clinicians should recognize that there are several standardized list-learning tests available to evaluate verbal memory. For example, an incomplete list of such tests includes the Rey Auditory-Verbal Learning Test (RAVLT),[26] California Verbal Learning Test (CVLT-II),[27] and Hopkins Verbal Learning Test (HVLT-Revised).[28] List-learning tasks are also frequently included in extended neuropsychological screening batteries and more comprehensive testing instruments (eg, Repeatable Battery for Assessment of Neuropsychological status [RBANS],[29,30] Wechsler Memory Scale [WMS][31,32]). While an individual with gross memory impairment is likely to perform in the impaired range across these different list-learning tests, there are subtle differences between tests that should be noted. For example, the CVLT-II list comprises words with semantic associations. The implication of this is that performance reflects an interaction of conceptual ability and verbal memory. It is debatable whether this is an advantage or a disadvantage. A recurrent finding in the literature is that individuals with left anterior temporal lobectomies show impaired recall of word lists.[33] Several list-learning tests include delayed recognition trials, which require a forced-choice decision as to whether a word was included on the original list. Because normative data suggest it is extremely unusual to observe multiple errors on a recognition trial, one-should carefully consider motivational factors before interpreting memory impairment.[34,35]

Wechsler Memory Scale

The Wechsler Memory Scale (WMS) has evolved over the years, from a relatively brief measure of immediate memory[36] to a more sophisticated instrument that evaluates auditory memory, visual memory, and visual working memory constructs.[32] The WMS-IV[32] includes primary subtests that require efficient encoding of short stories, word pairs, geometric figures, and the spatial location of abstract designs. Retention of this information is evaluated after an approximately 20-minute delay. An advantage of the WMS-IV over its predecessor is that more distinct dimensions of auditory and visual memory are evaluated.[37] The WMS-IV is arguably one of the most comprehensive memory tests available, but the trade-off is the extensive time required for administration and scoring.

Measures of Language Functioning

Western Aphasia Battery

The Western Aphasia Battery (WAB) is a comprehensive metric language evaluation tool that consists of 4 oral subtests (Spontaneous Speech; Auditory Comprehension; Repetition; Naming).[38] Performance on oral subtests is translated to an Aphasia Quotient (AQ) with normal (perfect) performance equal to a score of 100. Consideration of performance pattern and overall AQ can be used to determine the examinee's aphasia subtype (Broca, Wernicke, global, transcortical motor, transcortical sensory, transcortical mixed, anomic, or conduction). The WAB includes additional subtests that facilitate a more comprehensive understanding of communication abilities (Reading, Writing, Arithmetic, Gestural Praxis, Construction, Raven's Progressive Matrices). Additional subtest performances are combined to form a Performance Quotient (PQ), which may be combined with the AQ to derive a total summary score (Cortical Quotient; CQ). As might be anticipated, lower fluency, repetition, and confrontation naming scores were observed in individuals who had sustained left hemisphere stroke relative to individuals with mild forms of dementia.[39] Similar deficits are not generally observed in patients who sustain right hemisphere stroke.

Boston Naming Test

The Boston Naming Test (BNT) is a brief language test that requires an examinee to name 60 line drawings of objects that are increasingly difficult to identify.[40] If an examinee is unable to freely recall the name of an item, they are prompted with a phonemic cue after 20 seconds. The test is discontinued after 8 consecutive item failures. Fifteen-item and 30-item versions of the test have been developed, and generally function similarly to the original.[41,42] An individual's ability to complete this task is dependent on several factors such as age, education, vocabulary, and cultural background. There is compelling evidence that English language norms should not be used for bilingual speakers.[43] Poor performance on the BNT is not specific to a certain medical condition per se. A range of conditions such as cerebrovascular accident (most frequently to the left hemisphere), anoxia, small white matter infarcts in the brainstem, and subcortical disease such as multiple sclerosis or Parkinson disease may result in impaired BNT performance.[44]

Measures of Visuospatial Functioning

Rey-Osterrieth Complex Figure

The Rey-Osterrieth Complex Figure (ROCF) is a visuospatial constructional assessment tool that measures one's ability to conceptualize complex visual stimuli and to replicate accurate spatial orientation.[45] Common uses include not only the assessment of visuospatial perception and construction abilities but also visuospatial immediate and delayed memory recall abilities. In the Copy condition, patients are given a piece of paper and a pencil to reproduce a complex figure to the best of their ability. This test is not timed. However, the clinician may opt to further extend this assessment by testing the patient's ability to immediately recall the figure and then to recall the figure after a 30-minute delay. Performances are then scored using a 36-point scoring system, then compared with a demographically adjusted normative sample.[46]

Judgment of Line Orientation

The Judgment of Line Orientation (JLO) is a widely used, standardized measure of visuospatial judgment. This test measures one's ability to estimate angular orientations by visually matching angled line pairs to 11 numbered radii forming a semicircle.[47,48] There is also a randomized JLO with two 15-item short forms, which has good internal consistency and correlates well (0.94) with full score data.[48] This test can be used for purely visuospatial perception assessment, when motor dysfunction complicates test performance on copy tasks such as the ROCF.

Measures of Effort

Rey Fifteen-Item Test

The Rey Fifteen-Item Test (FIT) is a commonly used brief measure of task engagement.[26] It is suggested that anyone who is not significantly impaired can recall 9 of 15 items presented.[48] Clinicians should be cognizant that other interpretive cutoff scores have been proposed to differentiate between those putting forth adequate effort and those not. In general, adjusting a cutoff score upward will increase sensitivity at the expense of specificity. For the purpose of the test's integrity, details of the test provision are deliberately withheld from this article.

Test of Memory Malingering

The Test of Memory Malingering (TOMM) is a very effective instrument for detecting insufficient effort on neuropsychological measures. It does not appear that emotional status or physical functioning affects TOMM performance; if an examinee is engaged with testing it is expected that he or she will obtain perfect or nearly perfect scores.[48,49]

Of note, the TOMM has been used in clinical contexts involving chronic exposure to toxic agents.[12] For the purpose of the test's integrity, details of the test provision are deliberately withheld from this article.

Self-Report Measures

Emotional Intelligence Index

Some consider emotional intelligence as being more important than cognition in completing daily activities.[50] It reflects an individual's ability to respond adaptively and to competently cope with everyday difficulties. The Emotional Intelligence Index (EQ-I) is a self-report measure that evaluates EQ in 5 principal areas (Intrapersonal, Interpersonal, Stress Management, Adaptability, and General Mood). Each of these broad domains consists of 2 to 5 subcategories (eg, Interpersonal: Empathy, Social Responsibility, and Interpersonal Relationships). Interpretation of EQ-I scores are generally consistent with traditional cognitive intelligence measures. Given that there might be some uncertainty regarding interpretation of an emotional intelligence scale, the interpretive guideline for EQ-I scores is shown in **Table 1**.

Frontal Systems Behavioral Inventory

With respect to frontal network syndromes, a self-report neurobehavioral inventory such as the Frontal Systems Behavioral Inventory (FrSBe) may potentially complement performance-based measures in an efficient manner.[51,52] In general, clinicians should not be concerned if self-report and performance-based assessment diverges; the congruency between self-report and performance-based assessment is lower than might be anticipated.[53] There are several potential reasons why an individual might not exhibit quantifiable deficits on standardized performance-based tests (eg, the possibility that frontal network inefficiencies are not observed in structured testing environments). Requesting an individual to describe her or his typical experiences might more efficiently tap difficulties and result in improved clinical detection of dysexecutive issues. The FrSBe consists of two 46-item questionnaires. Individuals complete 5-point Likert-scale items that contribute to 3 domains of frontal functioning (Apathy, Disinhibition, Executive Function). A summary score is also calculated and observer forms are available. Normative data are provided in the Technical Manual. In general, T scores ranging from 50 to 60 are considered "normal" and those falling in a range between 60 and 65 are considered "borderline." A graphical output system is also available, which facilitates easy monitoring of symptoms and discussion of results.[3]

Table 1 The interpretive guideline for EQ-I	
Interpretive Guideline	**Standard Score**
Markedly high: atypical well developed emotional capacity	>130
Very high: extremely well developed emotional capacity	120–129
High, well developed emotional capacity	110–119
Average: adequate emotional capacity	90–109
Low: underdeveloped emotional capacity	80–89
Very low: extremely underdeveloped emotional capacity	70–79
Markedly low: atypically impaired emotional capacity	<70

Extended Global Neurocognitive Screen

Repeatable Battery for Assessment of Neuropsychological Status

The Repeatable Battery for Assessment of Neuropsychological Status (RBANS) is an easy to administer and popular screening battery of global neuropsychological status.[3,29] After about 30 minutes of testing, a standardized score for each cognitive domain is produced, that is, Immediate Memory, Visuospatial/Constructional, Language, Attention, Delayed Memory, and a Total Scale Score of neuropsychological status. Another positive aspect of this test is that the screening battery is repeatable with an alternative form. The trade-off for this and efficiency in time for administration is that the sensitivity and specificity are sacrificed as compared with a more extended and comprehensive battery.

SUMMARY

This article aims to highlight some commonly used neuropsychological measures as used in the clinical management of neurotoxic exposure. As neurotoxic exposure can manifest in many different ways cognitively, it is important to have an approach that can assess all cognitive domains with efficiency. Unfortunately, this can be further complicated if the patient provides suboptimal effort regardless of the etiology, for example, malingering for secondary gain versus fatigue versus inattention as a true clinical manifestation. Accordingly, a formal effort measure may be useful, especially when management of toxic exposure involves potential litigation and secondary gain for parties involved. As for global cognitive deficits after exposure, it is critical to use a true multidisciplinary approach in patient care, involving the attending provider, neuropsychologist, physical therapist, occupational therapist, and social worker, to name a few. This approach may facilitate an easier transition for the patient to a more fruitful cognitive rehabilitation.

REFERENCES

1. Hartman DE. Neuropsychological toxicology: identification and assessment of human neurotoxic syndromes. 1st edition. New York: Pergamon Press; 1988.
2. Grandjean P, Landrigan PJ. Developmental neurotoxicity of industrial chemicals. Lancet 2006;368(9553):2167–78.
3. Dobbs MR. Clinical neurotoxicology: syndromes, substances, environments. Philadelphia: Saunders/Elsevier; 2009.
4. Freed DM, Kandel E. Long-term occupational exposure and the diagnosis of dementia. Neurotoxicology 1988;9(3):391–400.
5. Kukull WA, Larson EB, Bowen JD, et al. Solvent exposure as a risk factor for Alzheimer's disease: a case-control study. Am J Epidemiol 1995;141(11):1059–71 [discussion: 1072–9].
6. Isbister GK, Buckley NA, Whyte IM. Serotonin toxicity: a practical approach to diagnosis and treatment. Med J Aust 2007;187(6):361–5.
7. Eubig PA, Aguiar A, Schantz SL. Lead and PCBs as risk factors for attention deficit/hyperactivity disorder. Environ Health Perspect 2010;118(12):1654–67.
8. Kuehn BM. Increased risk of ADHD associated with early exposure to pesticides, PCBs. JAMA 2010;304(1):27–8.
9. Assessment: neuropsychological testing of adults. Considerations for neurologists. Report of the Therapeutics and Technology Assessment Subcommittee of the American Academy of Neurology. Neurology 1996;47(2):592–9.

10. Faust D, Hart K, Guilmette TJ, et al. Neuropsychologists capacity to detect adolescent malingerers. Prof Psychol Res Pr 1988;19(5):508–15.
11. Heaton RK, Smith HH, Lehman RA, et al. Prospects for faking believable deficits on neuropsychological testing. J Consult Clin Psychol 1978;46(5): 892–900.
12. van Hout MSE, Schmand B, Wekking EM, et al. Suboptimal performance on neuropsychological tests in patients with suspected chronic toxic encephalopathy. Neurotoxicology 2003;24(4/5):547–51.
13. Lamberty GJ, Putnam SH, Chatel DM, et al. Derived trail making test indices: a preliminary-report. Neuropsychiatry, Neuropsychology, & Behavioral Neurology 1994;7(3):230–4.
14. Stroop JR. Studies of interference in serial verbal reactions [PhD]. Nashville (TN): George Peabody College for Teachers; 1935.
15. Mitrushina MN. Handbook of normative data for neuropsychological assessment. 2nd edition. New York: Oxford University Press; 2005.
16. Ternerry MR, Corsson B, DeBoe J, et al. Visual search and attention test. Lutz (FL): Psychological Assessment Resources, Inc; 1990.
17. Heaton RK, Psychological Assessment Resources Inc. WCST-CV4. Computer 4, research edition. Lutz (FL): Psychological Assessment Resources; 2003.
18. Rhodes MG. Age-related differences in performance on the Wisconsin Card Sorting Test: a meta-analytic review. Psychol Aging 2004;19(3):482–94.
19. Larrabee GJ. Detection of malingering using atypical performance patterns on standard neuropsychological tests. Clin Neuropsychol 2003;17(3):410–25.
20. Delis DC, Kaplan E, Kramer JH. Delis-Kaplan executive function system technical manual. San Antonio (TX): Pearson; 2001.
21. Culbertson WC, Zillmer EA. TOLDX 2nd edition: Tower of LondonDX 2nd edition. North Tonawanda (NY): Multi-Health Systems; 2001.
22. Samet MG, Marshall-Mies JC. Expanded Complex Cognitive Assessment Battery (CCAB): final test administrator user guide. Alexandria (VA): System Research Laboratory: U.S. Army Research Institute; 1987.
23. Goel V, Grafman J. Are the frontal lobes implicated in planning functions—interpreting data from the Tower-of-Hanoi. Neuropsychologia 1995;33(5):623–42.
24. Carlin D, Bonerba J, Phipps M, et al. Planning impairments in frontal lobe dementia and frontal lobe lesion patients. Neuropsychologia 2000;38(5):655–65.
25. Lazeron RH, Rombouts SA, Machielsen WC, et al. Visualizing brain activation during planning: the Tower of London test adapted for functional MR imaging. AJNR Am J Neuroradiol 2000;21(8):1407–14.
26. Rey A. L'examen clinique en psychologie. Paris: Presses Universitarires de France; 1964 [in French].
27. Delis DC, Kramer JH, Kaplan E, et al. California verbal learning test—second edition (CVLT-II). San Antonio (TX): Pearson; 2000.
28. Benedict RHB, Schretlen D, Groninger L, et al. Hopkins Verbal Learning Test Revised: normative data and analysis of inter-form and test-retest reliability. Clin Neuropsychol 1998;12(1):43–55.
29. Randolph C. Repeatable Battery for the Assessment of Neuropsychological Status (RBANS). San Antonio (TX): Pearson; 1998.
30. Randolph C, Tierney MC, Mohr E, et al. The Repeatable Battery for the Assessment of Neuropsychological Status (RBANS): preliminary clinical validity. J Clin Exp Neuropsychol 1998;20(3):310–9.
31. Wechsler D. Wechsler Memory Scale—third edition (WMS-III). San Antonio (TX): The Psychological Corporation; 1997.

32. Wechsler D. Wechsler Memory Scale—fourth edition (WMS-IV). San Antonio (TX): Pearson; 2009.
33. Majdan A, Sziklas V, JonesGotman M. Performance of healthy subjects and patients with resection from the anterior temporal lobe on matched tests of verbal and visuoperceptual learning. J Clin Exp Neuropsychol 1996;18(3):416–30.
34. Mitrushina MN, Boone KB, D'Elia L. Handbook of normative data for neuropsychological assessment. New York: Oxford University Press; 1999.
35. Schmidt M. Rey auditory verbal learning test. A handbook. Los Angeles (CA): Western Psychological Services; 1996.
36. Wechsler DA. Standardized memory scale for clinical use. J Psychol 1945;19: 87–95.
37. Hoelzle JB, Nelson NW, Smith CA. Comparison of Wechsler Memory Scale—fourth edition (WMS-IV) and third edition (WMS-III) dimensional structures: improved ability to evaluate auditory and visual constructs. J Clin Exp Neuropsychol 2011;33(3):283–91.
38. Kertesz A. The western aphasia battery revised. San Antonio (TX): Pearson; 2007.
39. Horner J, Dawson DV, Heyman A, et al. The usefulness of the Western Aphasia Battery for differential diagnosis of Alzheimer dementia and focal stroke syndromes—preliminary evidence. Brain Lang 1992;42(1):77–88.
40. Kaplan E, Goodglass H, Barresi B. Boston naming test. 2nd edition. Lippincott, Williams, Wilkins; 2001.
41. Morris JC, Heyman A, Mohs RC, et al. The Consortium to Establish a Registry for Alzheimers-Disease (CERAD). 1. Clinical and neuropsychological assessment of Alzheimers disease. Neurology 1989;39(9):1159–65.
42. Williams BW, Mack W, Henderson VW. Boston Naming Test in Alzheimers disease. Neuropsychologia 1989;27(8):1073–9.
43. Roberts PM, Garcia LJ, Desrochers A, et al. English performance of proficient bilingual adults on the Boston Naming Test. Aphasiology 2002;16(4–6):11p.
44. Strauss E, Sherman EMS, Spreen O. A compendium of neuropsychological tests: administration, norms, and commentary. Oxford. 3rd edition. New York: Oxford University Press; 2006.
45. Osterrieth PA. Filetest de copie d'une figure complex: contribution a l'etude de la perception et de la memoire. Archives de Psychologie 1944;30:286–356 [in French].
46. Meyers JE, Meyers KR. Rey complex figure test and recognition trial. Lutz (FL): Psychological Assessment Resources, Inc; 2002.
47. Benton AL, Sivan AB, Hamsher K. Judgment of line orientation. Lutz (FL): Psychological Assessment Resources; 1994.
48. Lezak MD. Neuropsychological assessment. Oxford. 4th edition. New York: Oxford University Press; 2004.
49. Tombaugh TN. Test of memory malingering. San Antonio (TX): Pearson Education, Inc; 1996.
50. Bar-On R. EQ-I: Emotional Quotient-Inventory. Toronto: Multi-Health Systems; 2001.
51. Grace J, Malloy P, Psychological Assessment Resources Inc. FrSBe, frontal systems behavior scale: professional manual. Lutz (FL): Psychological Assessment Resources; 2001.
52. Mesulam MM. Principles of behavioral and cognitive neurology. Oxford. 2nd edition. New York: Oxford University Press; 2000.
53. Meyer GJ, Finn SE, Eyde LD, et al. Psychological testing and psychological assessment—a review of evidence and issues. Am Psychol 2001;56(2):128–65.

Toxic Leukoencephalopathies

Laura M. Tormoehlen, MD[a,b,*]

KEYWORDS

- Post-anoxic • Carbon monoxide
- Delayed neurologic sequelae • Heroin • "Chasing the dragon"
- Posterior reversible encephalopathy syndrome

Leukoencephalopathy is a syndrome of neurologic deficits, including alteration of mental status, caused by pathologic changes in the cerebral white matter. The term, *toxic leukoencephalopathy*, encompasses a wide variety of exposures and clinical presentations. The MRI findings in each of these entities is similar given the requisite involvement of the cerebral white matter but may be quite different in the distribution of areas involved, the extent of gray matter involvement, and findings on ancillary radiographic studies. The diagnosis in these syndromes is made by careful attention to the history, clinical features, and radiologic findings. The differential diagnosis of toxin-induced leukoencephalopathy includes multiple sclerosis, acute disseminated encephalomyelitis, progressive multifocal leukoencephalopathy, several rare leukodystrophies, gliomatosis cerebri, and encephalitis. The goal of this article is to give a detailed discussion of three of the best-defined toxic leukoencephalopathies: delayed posthypoxic leukoencephalopathy (DPHL), including delayed neurologic sequelae (DNS) of carbon monoxide (CO) poisoning; heroin inhalation leukoencephalopathy; and posterior reversible encephalopathy syndrome (PRES).

DELAYED POSTHYPOXIC LEUKOENCEPHALOPATHY

DPHL is a rare demyelinating syndrome that may occur after a prolonged period of poor cerebral oxygenation. The usual presentation is characterized by complete or near-complete recovery from the acute event, followed by onset of neuropsychologic symptoms days to weeks later. This pattern of symptomatology distinguishes it from acute hypoxic brain injury, which results in persistent effects and is associated with greater involvement of the gray matter.

The author has nothing to disclose.

[a] Department of Neurology, Indiana University School of Medicine, 545 Barnhill Drive, Indianapolis, IN 46202, USA

[b] Department of Emergency Medicine, Indiana University School of Medicine, 1701 North Senate Boulevard B401, Indianapolis, IN 46202, USA

* 1701 North Senate Boulevard, B417, Indianapolis, IN 46202.

E-mail address: laumjone@iupui.edu

Neurol Clin 29 (2011) 591–605

doi:10.1016/j.ncl.2011.05.005

0733-8619/11/$ – see front matter © 2011 Elsevier Inc. All rights reserved.

neurologic.theclinics.com

Clinical Features

This phenomenon was first described in cases of CO toxicity[1] but has now been described in cases of cardiac arrest, complications of surgery and anesthesia, asphyxial gas poisoning, strangulation, shock, and respiratory depression from heroin or benzodiazepine overdose.[2–9]

Historically, DPHL is heralded by an acute event resulting in hypoxic insult. In all cases that are not associated with CO (discussed later), there is a period of unconsciousness or coma.[10] This is followed by neurologic recovery with subsequent return to usual activities. Then, after a period of days to weeks, there is acute deterioration with onset of neuropsychiatric symptoms that worsen over the course of a few days. Symptoms may include akinetic mutism (apathy, incontinence, mutism, and pseudobulbar affect) or parkinsonian features (tremor, gait and speech disturbance, rigidity, and masked facies), suggesting involvement of the white matter tracts of the frontal lobes and basal ganglia motor circuits, respectively.[2,11]

Radiologic Findings

Diffuse, confluent hypodensity of the white matter on CT of the head can be diagnostic if the clinical history suggests the possibility of DPHL. If the history is not clear or other diagnoses are possible, MRI is necessary to entertain the diagnosis. Classic MRI findings are T2-sequence hyperintense lesions in the periventricular white matter of the cerebral hemispheres with relative sparing of the cerebellum and brainstem. The lesions are typically nonenhancing and do not extend into the cortex. MR spectroscopy in DPHL patients has been reported to show an elevated choline peak, indicative of lipid membrane turnover and suggestive of demyelination.[12,13]

Pathophysiology and Pathologic Findings

The clinical event preceding DPHL produces a mild-to-moderate hypoxia. Severe hypoxia is more likely to result in acute, persistent hypoxic brain injury. Because the gray matter is more susceptible to acute severe hypoxia, the acute brain injury is characterized by lesions in the basal ganglia and cortex. A less severe episode of hypoxia may allow initial neurologic recovery followed by the pathologic demyelination characteristic of DPHL. Microscopic examination reveals severe diffuse demyelination with axonal sparing. Reactive astrocytes and macrophages are present, and there is no evidence of intramyelinic vacuolization, thus distinguishing it from heroin inhalation leukoencephalopathy.[4,13]

Although there are many diverse causes of cerebral hypoxia, they are categorized into 4 mechanisms in *Plum and Posner's Diagnosis of Stupor and Coma*[14]: hypoxic hypoxia (low oxygen tension: high altitudes and asphyxial gases), anemic hypoxia (decreased oxygen carrying capacity: anemia and hemoglobinopathy), ischemic hypoxia (insufficient cerebral blood flow: shock, myocardial infarction, and stroke), and histotoxic hypoxia (mitochondrial toxins: cyanide and CO). All 4 mechanisms are equally capable of producing insufficient oxygenation of the brain tissue.[14]

The exact mechanism of the delayed-onset leukoencephalopathy is not yet clear. One theory suggests that hypoxia/hypoperfusion induces necrosis of the oligodendroglia in the border zones between cerebral vascular territories.[15] The delayed onset of symptoms is then due to the time between oligodendroglial injury and loss of myelin.[2] If this were the isolated mechanism, however, DPHL should be much more common. The infrequency of DPHL indicates the possibility of a requisite genetic susceptibility. Some investigators have proposed pseudodeficiency of arylsulfatase A as a predisposing condition[7,13]; however, cases of DPHL with normal arylsulfatase

A levels have been reported.[2,15,16] Thus, although pseudodeficiency of arylsulfatase A may predispose to DPHL, it is not a prerequisite condition. There may be other enzyme deficiencies with similar effect or additional undiscovered predisposing conditions.

Heroin use has been associated with DPHL in the setting of associated respiratory depression and hypoxia. Heroin pyrolysate (vapor) likely has additional mechanisms of toxicity and produces a clinical syndrome of "chasing the dragon" leukoencephalopathy that is distinct from DPHL by radiologic and pathologic findings (discussed later).

Treatment and Prognosis

Aggressive supportive care is the core of treatment. No effective pharmaceutical or interventional therapy is known. An unsuccessful trial of immunomodulatory therapy (high-dose steroids and plasmapheresis) has been reported in DPHL after ethanol and morphine intoxication.[17] Otherwise, there are no available data on specific treatment of this condition.

There are limited data on the prognosis of patients who develop DPHL that is not related to CO exposure. Although death has been reported,[17] most patients experience some functional recovery with variable degrees of persistent cognitive and neurologic deficits.[2,4,7,9,13,15,16,18] Neurorehabilitation with multimodality therapies is essential for continued recovery.[10]

Delayed Leukoencephalopathy of Carbon Monoxide Toxicity

The delayed leukoencephalopathy of acute CO toxicity is a subtype of DPHL. There are, however, clinical features and pathologic mechanisms that make this a distinct clinical entity. This is the group of patients with DPHL that are the best defined in the literature. In 1983, Choi published a large case series of 2360 patients with acute CO toxicity.[1] DNS were diagnosed in 65 cases (2.75%) with a mean lucid interval of 22.4 days (range 2–40 days).[1]

Characteristic clinical features of DNS include memory and cognitive deficits, apathy, mutism, urinary incontinence, and gait disturbance. Signs referable to the frontal lobe (primitive reflexes) and basal ganglia (masked facies and rigidity) are common, whereas cerebellar signs are uncommon. Incidence of delayed symptoms seems to increase with the duration of unconsciousness from acute toxicity. The sequelae can occur in patients who had retained consciousness during the acute intoxication, however. In 2 case series with more than 3000 patients with acute CO toxicity, DNS did not occur in any patient under the age of 30 years,[1,19] suggesting an increased susceptibility in older adults.

The MRI findings in delayed leukoencephalopathy after acute CO toxicity are the same as those in DPHL. Acutely, there may be lesions in the basal ganglia on MRI, likely reflective of a more severe event and the susceptibility of the basal ganglia to hypoxia and hypotension induced by cellular asphyxiants. These are usually characterized by T2-sequence hyperintensity that may persist on the MRI done for the delayed symptoms (**Fig. 1**).[20,21] Single photon-emission CT (SPECT) in patients with DNS reveals diffuse, patchy hypoperfusion throughout the cerebral cortex, and some patients show a correlation between improvement in perfusion and clinical improvement.[22,23]

Although the mechanism of inadequate oxygen supply in DPHL may be any or a combination of the first 3 of *Plum and Posner's* mechanisms (hypoxic, anemic, or ischemic), CO toxicity also causes histotoxic hypoxia.[14] CO causes cellular hypoxia by replacing oxyhemoglobin with carboxyhemoglobin, resulting in a functional anemia, and shifting the oxygen-dissociation curve to the left, resulting in decreased oxygen delivery. This mechanism alone, however, is not sufficient to explain toxicity. In both animal and human studies, the level of carboxyhemoglobin in the blood

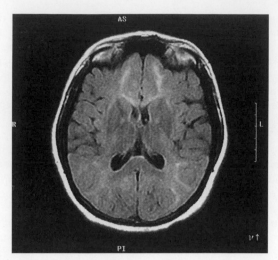

Fig. 1. DPHL in a 46-year-old woman after recovery from acute CO toxicity 3 weeks prior. The bilateral basal ganglia lesions were present on MRI performed on day 3 after acute CO toxicity. The MRI above was performed 6 days after the onset of pseudobulbar affect, confusion, and memory loss. It shows FLAIR hyperintense lesions in the periventricular white matter of both hemispheres.

correlates poorly with the severity of clinical effects.[24,25] CO is a direct cellular toxin via binding to cytochromes, resulting in disruption of oxidative metabolism. It also seems to increase nitric oxide levels leading to oxygen-free radical production. This then may initiate a cascade of events starting with activation of intravascular neutrophils and culminating in brain lipid peroxidation.[26,27]

Treatment of DNS, once it has occurred, is supportive care. Certainly, the standard of care in the setting of acute CO poisoning is high-flow oxygen to treat hypoxia and enhance elimination of CO. There is, however, much debate about the use of hyperbaric oxygen therapy (HBOT) to prevent DNS. To date, 7 prospective randomized controlled trials have compared HBOT with normobaric oxygen for acute CO poisoning.[28–34] Four studies show a benefit of HBOT over normobaric oxygen and 3 do not. Differences in HBOT protocols and outcome measures make definitive conclusions difficult. In general, HBOT is recommended for patients with loss of consciousness, altered mental status, focal neurologic deficits, cardiovascular dysfunction, or severe metabolic acidosis.[35] HBOT is also recommended for pregnant women with CO-hemoglobin levels greater than 15% to 20%, due to the tight binding of CO to fetal hemoglobin. Those patients not meeting these criteria for HBOT should receive normobaric oxygen at 100% by tight-fitting face mask for 6 to 12 hours.[26] The prognosis of DNS is good, with recovery or near-recovery in 61% to 75% of patients within 1 year.[1,19]

HEROIN INHALATION LEUKOENCEPHALOPATHY

The smoking of heroin is a practice that began in Shanghai in the 1920s. "Chasing the dragon" is a method of smoking heroin, born in Hong Kong in the 1950s, that involves inhalation of the vapor (pyrolysate) of heated heroin, typically by using a flame to heat the heroin on folded aluminium foil. Because the hydrochloride form of heroin has become less available over time, it has been replaced by the freebase form. Although the hydrochloride is more easily dissolved in water for injection, the freebase form of heroin is poorly soluble in water but sublimates easily when heated. Thus, chasing the dragon as a technique has become more prevalent because of the availability of the freebase form of heroin as well as the safety concerns surrounding injection methods.[36] The bioavailability of inhaling the vapors of heated heroin is good,[37] especially when in the base form, and may be augmented by the presence of caffeine or barbiturates.[36]

Clinical Features

The first cases of heroin pyrolysate–induced leukoencephalopathy were described by Wolters and colleagues[38] in 1982. The clinical syndrome is characterized by 3 stages, through which each patient may or may not progress. The first stage manifests as a primarily cerebellar syndrome with gait and limb ataxia, soft pseudobulbar speech, apathy, and akathisia. In the second stage, worsening ataxia, spastic paresis, choreoathetoid movements, and myoclonus may occur. Primitive reflexes (palmomental, snout, and oculomandibular) may also emerge in this stage. The terminal stage is characterized by hyperpyrexia, hypotonic paresis, akinetic mutism, and stretching spasms.[38,39] Long and colleagues[40] describe these stretching spasms as "opisthotonic and decerebrate-like posturing."

Progression through these stages occurs over weeks to months.[37,41,42] Of Wolters and colleagues'[38] 47 patients, 26 progressed to the second stage and 11 reached the third, terminal stage. The diagnosis is made on the basis of clinical and imaging features: history of heroin inhalation, cerebellar syndrome, and symmetric white matter lesions of the cerebellum and posterior cerebrum. A recent case series of 27 patients from British Columbia included 1 case of mild symptoms after a single use; all others had used heroin by inhalation for 3 years or more.[42] Some of the cases report the onset of symptoms coinciding with heroin withdrawal,[43,44] whereas others describe onset of symptoms during continued heroin use.[44–48]

Radiologic Findings

The classic findings on MRI include abnormally high T2 signal in symmetric distribution in the cerebellar and posterior cerebral hemispheres, including the posterior limbs of the internal capsule (**Fig. 2**).[39,41,45,49,50] There is relative sparing of the dentate nuclei in the cerebellum, the subcortical U-fibers in the posterior cerebrum, and the anterior limbs of the internal capsules as well as the gray matter in general.[41,46,49] Other reported areas of cerebral involvement include bilateral hippocampi and basal ganglia,[45] thalami,[51] and the corpus callosum.[41,50,52] Reported areas of brainstem involvement include the superior cerebellar peduncles,[38,43] medial lemniscus,[49,50,52] and pyramidal tracts.[49,50,52] Cases that have reported normal signal in the cerebellum

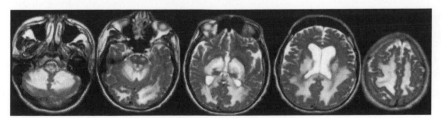

Fig. 2. Chasing the dragon leukoencephalopathy in a 24-year-old man. T2-weighted images of the brain show hyperintense signal in the cerebellum, brainstem, posterior limbs of the internal capsules, thalami, and occipital lobes. (*From* Bartlett E, Mikulis DJ. Chasing "chasing the dragon" with MRI: leukoencephalopathy in drug abuse. Br J Radiol 2005;78:997–1004; with permission.)

either involved intravenous use of heroin or did not establish clear evidence of heroin inhalation.[53–55]

The MRI lesions do not enhance with contrast[39,50] and are typically not diffusion restricted, although diffusion restriction has been reported on MRI performed early in the clinical course when the cellular damage is likely ongoing.[50] Magnetic resonance (MR) spectroscopy demonstrates a reduced N-acetylaspartate peak and an inverted lactate doublet[50,56] with a normal or reduced choline peak.[51] N-acetylaspartate is a marker of neuronal integrity, so the reduction may be secondary to either axonal injury or mitochondrial damage. Choline elevation occurs with demyelination, and the absence of this finding supports the conclusion that demyelination does not occur in this condition. The inverted lactate doublet indicates increased brain lactate content, which suggests conversion to anaerobic metabolism. This constellation of findings on MR spectroscopy is most consistent with mitochondrial dysfunction.[39,41,51,56]

Pathophysiology and Pathologic Findings

Because the classic chasing the dragon leukoencephalopathy does not typically occur with other methods of heroin use, the etiology is most likely related to the method of preparation or a contaminant of the heroin used for inhalation. Triethyltin can be formed from inorganic tin under some conditions and is known to cause a myelinopathy. Tests on commonly available aluminum foil have not demonstrated levels of tin high enough to account for the clinical syndrome.[41] Evaluations of street heroin samples have revealed only known contaminants and cutting agents,[36,42,57,58] none of which is particularly neurotoxic. The rarity of this complication and the occurrence of small epidemics imply that if a contaminant is the cause, it is one added sporadically at the end of the production process.[42] In addition, leukoencephalopathy does not reliably occur in all persons exposed to the same heroin at the same time,[41,47] suggesting the possibility of a required genetic predisposition. Because of the pathologic findings of vacuolar myelinopathy, it is expected that the etiologic toxin is lipophilic[46]; however, the exact cause of this condition remains elusive.

Gross neuropathologic evaluation reveals significant edema. Microscopically, spongiform degeneration of the white matter, characterized by vacuolization within the myelin, is apparent.[59,60] The vacuoles may be so abundant as to coalesce into larger voids.[38] There is reduction in the number of oligodendrocytes without evidence of myelin breakdown products.[59] Axonal degeneration with vacuolar degeneration and mitochondrial swelling may be present as well.[38] Gray matter is unaffected as are the subcortical U-fibers, spinal cord, and peripheral nerves. The pathologic changes usually seen after severe hypoxia, including ischemia-induced neuronal changes and vascular congestion, are notably absent.[40,44,58,59]

Creutzfeldt-Jakob disease is a prion-induced spongiform degeneration that largely affects gray matter. Other causes of spongiform leukoencephalopathy are triethyltin, hexachlorophene, actinomycin D, isonicotinic acid, hydrazine, cycloleucine, cuprizone, and ethidium bromide.[41]

Treatment and Prognosis

The mortality rate in the original case series of 47 patients was 23%.[38] A recent case series of 27 patients reports a mortality rate of 48%.[42] The rarity of this disease process precludes prospective studies to determine risk factors and treatment for heroin pyrolysate-induced spongiform leukoencephalopathy. The features of MR spectroscopy and neuropathology findings support the hypothesis that mitochondrial dysfunction is a contributor to the pathophysiology. Some authors report improvement in symptoms after treatment with an antioxidant drug regimen of ubiquinone (coenzyme Q), vitamin C, and vitamin E.[41,48] Given the favorable side-effect profile of this drug combination, treatment should be considered when the diagnosis is made.

POSTERIOR REVERSIBLE ENCEPHALOPATHY SYNDROME

PRES is a condition with many names. First described as reversible posterior leukoencephalopathy syndrome in 1996, it is a clinicoradiologic diagnosis that is associated with an ever-growing number of medical conditions. It has been called reversible posterior cerebral edema syndrome, hyperperfusion encephalopathy, and brain capillary leak syndrome, but is now commonly titled PRES. Although PRES accurately describes the typical clinical presentation and radiologic findings, some dispute this title because cerebral involvement is not always confined to the territory of the posterior circulation. Severe cases may have areas of cerebral infarction or hemorrhage; thus, the condition is not always reversible. It is perhaps appropriate that it is no longer termed a leukoencephalopathy because the gray matter is often involved, albeit to a lesser extent, and this is frequently manifested by seizures.

In the original case series of 15 patients by Hinchey and colleagues[61] in 1996, 8 were on immunosuppressive therapy, 3 had eclampsia, and 4 had renal disease. Of these patients, 12 had acute hypertension and 11 had seizures. The medical conditions that have a well-established association with PRES are hypertension, eclampsia, autoimmune disease, sepsis/shock, cancer chemotherapy, immunosuppressive therapy, and transplantation.[62] The occurrence of the cerebral vasogenic edema that typifies PRES in this plethora of disease states makes the determination of its pathogenesis complex. This discussion focuses on toxin-induced PRES (ie, immunosuppressive and chemotherapeutic agents).

Clinical Features

The range of clinical symptoms caused by PRES is varied but typically includes headache, encephalopathy, nausea, and vision loss. Signs and symptoms may develop over hours to days. Seizures may occur at the onset of symptoms or later in the course. Moderate-to-severe hypertension is present in 70% to 80% of patients; the remainder have mild hypertension or normal blood pressure.[61,63] Cranial nerve deficits may occur but are rare. The diagnosis of PRES is made by the clinical history, neurologic examination, and neuroimaging. The presence of pre-existing conditions, including pregnancy or recent delivery, acute hypertension, autoimmune conditions, renal disease, or cytotoxic therapy, is supportive of the diagnosis. Differential diagnosis includes ischemic or hemorrhagic stroke, subarachnoid hemorrhage, venous sinus thrombosis, obstructive hydrocephalus, encephalitis, vasculitis, and central demyelination syndromes (acute disseminated encephalomyelitis and central pontine myelinolysis).

The immunosuppressive drugs that are most commonly associated with PRES are the calcineurin inhibitors, cyclosporine and tacrolimus. It has also been reported with bevacizumab, interferon, methotrexate, rituximab, sirolimus, sorafenib, sunitinib, fingolimod, and intravenous immunoglobulin.[61,64–76] The chemotherapeutic agents linked with PRES are cisplatin, cytarabine, doxorubicin, cyclophosphamide, gemcitabine, vincristine, and etoposide.[65,77–82] Drug levels do not seem to correlate with development of PRES, as it has been reported to develop in patients with therapeutic levels of both cyclosporine and tacrolimus.[81,83] The route of administration may also be a factor in the development of PRES. For example, intrathecal administration of methotrexate seems to be associated with a higher incidence of PRES than the intravenous route.[84,85] Fluid overload, mild hypertension, and renal dysfunction are also considered risk factors for the development of PRES.[80]

According to a large case series of 4222 patients, the incidence of PRES after solid-organ transplant is 0.49% (21 cases) without a difference between transplant types.[86] An additional 6 cases were reported outside of the study period for a total of 27 cases, and 7 of these 27 cases presented with an isolated seizure. The remaining 20 patients presented with a combination of headache, encephalopathy, and vision change; 12 of these went on to have a seizure. Blood pressure was normal in 8, mildly elevated in 6, and severely elevated in 13.[86] The timing of onset was more likely to be early (within 2 months of transplant) for liver transplantation and later (1 year or longer after transplant) for kidney transplantation. There are few data on the incidence of PRES with specific drugs, although small case series have reported a 1.6% incidence of tacrolimus-associated PRES and a 7.5% incidence of cyclosporin A–associated PRES in hematopoietic stem cell transplant patients.[87,88]

Radiologic Findings

Neuroimaging typically reveals evidence of white matter edema with symmetric involvement of the occipitoparietal regions (**Fig. 3**).[61,63,89,90] Although vasogenic edema is the hallmark of PRES, cases with areas of cytotoxic edema suggestive of focal infarction have been described.[91–93] Thus, although CT usually depicts hypodense lesions in the affected regions, MRI is the diagnostic test of choice because of the utility of diffusion-weighted imaging (DWI) in differentiating vasogenic from cytotoxic edema. Identification of the affected cortical and subcortical areas is best performed by the fluid-attenuated inversion recovery (FLAIR) sequence.[94] Then, DWI and apparent diffusion coefficient (ADC) mapping allow assessment of the type of edema: vasogenic (isointense or hyperintense on DWI and hyperintense on ADC) versus cytotoxic (hyperintense on DWI and hypointense on ADC).[92,93,95]

The classic pattern of involvement in PRES is bilateral and symmetric lesions in the cortex and subcortical white matter of the occipital and parietal lobes. Lesions in the posterior frontal and temporal lobes as well as the cerebellum, brainstem, thalamus, and basal ganglia are increasingly reported.[91] An MRI pattern involving these areas has been termed, atypical PRES, but is likely more common than previously recognized. Although there may be lesions in areas not supplied by the posterior circulation, the predominant MRI findings are posterior. Serial imaging demonstrates improvement or resolution in most cases.

MR angiography demonstrates findings of diffuse vasoconstriction or focal vasoconstriction alternating with vasodilation, consistent with vasospasm.[96–101] Catheter

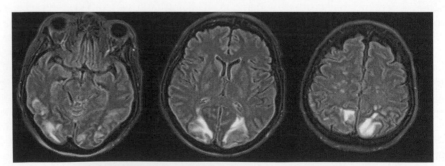

Fig. 3. PRES in a 54-year-old woman who presented with altered mental status, seizures, and vision changes while taking tacrolimus for immunosuppression after liver transplantation. FLAIR images show hyperintensity in the bilateral occipital lobes. She clinically improved after immunosuppression was changed from tacrolimus to cyclosporine.

angiography in patients with PRES reveals similar findings.[99,102–106] Single-photon emission CT (SPECT) results have been less consistent in that some studies have reported hyperperfusion on SPECT and some have reported hypoperfusion.[90,107–109]

Pathophysiology and Pathologic Findings

The origin of PRES is complex and controversial. Vasogenic edema in the subcortical white matter of the posterior circulation, with variable involvement of the cortex and the territory of the anterior circulation, is the accepted cause of symptoms. It is the etiology of the edema that is currently under debate. The hyperperfusion theory holds that abnormal autoregulation allows for increased perfusion in the setting of hypertension, resulting in breakdown of the blood-brain barrier and vasogenic edema.[61,80,90] The relatively reduced number of adrenergic nerves in the vertebrobasilar circulation may predispose this region to the development of edema.[110,111] Alternatively, vasoconstriction, as a normal autoregulatory response to hypertension, leads to hypoperfusion followed by ischemia and vasogenic edema.[112] Endothelial dysfunction, whether from an immunologic process or direct drug toxicity, likely plays a role in pathogenesis as well.[61,75,112]

During the acute phase, pathologic findings on microscopy are consistent with vasogenic edema. Reactive astrocytes with macrophages and lymphocytes have been observed, usually without evidence of inflammation or neuronal damage.[83,113–115] Histopathologic findings on autopsy specimen after a prolonged course demonstrate necrotic foci and other features consistent with ischemia.[81–83,116]

Treatment and Prognosis

Diagnosis of PRES is the initial step in treatment because recognition of the pathologic process leads to identification of etiologic factors. Removal of causative agents, treatment of seizures, and measured lowering of blood pressure are the mainstay of treatment. Transplant patients who require immunosuppression may improve with transition to another immunosuppressive agent or a decrease in the dose.[62] Prognosis is usually good, with recovery over the course of days, after appropriate care is initiated.[61] Delay in diagnosis can result in progression of the edema and may contribute to permanent neurologic sequelae from cerebral infarction or hemorrhage.[95,96] Death is a rarely reported complication.[116,117]

SUMMARY

Leukoencephalopathy is a clinical and radiologic diagnosis with a wide variety of causes, including infections, autoimmune disease, neoplasms, and metabolic disorders as well as many toxins not addressed in this article (eg, radiation, ethanol, and toluene).

DPHL is characterized by recovery from a recent hypoxic event followed by acute onset of neuropsychiatric symptoms. MRI findings include T2-sequence hyperintense lesions in the periventricular white matter of both hemispheres, usually involving the frontal lobes and sparing the cerebellum and brainstem. Treatment is supportive care.

Heroin inhalation leukoencephalopathy usually presents as a cerebellar syndrome in the setting of chronic inhalation of heroin vapor (chasing the dragon). MRI findings include symmetric T2-sequence hyperintense lesions in the cerebellum and posterior cerebral hemispheres. Pathologic evaluation demonstrates intramyelinic vacuolization. Treatment is largely supportive care, although antioxidant therapy may be considered.

PRES is characterized by headache, vision changes, seizures, and alteration of mental status. This may occur in the setting of acute hypertension, eclampsia, autoimmune disease, sepsis/shock, cancer chemotherapy, immunosuppressive therapy, and transplantation. MRI findings include T2-sequence hyperintense lesions in the occipitoparietal regions. Removal of causative medications as well as the treatment of seizures and hypertension is the appropriate treatment regimen.

REFERENCES

1. Choi IS. Delayed neurologic sequelae in carbon monoxide intoxication. Arch Neurol 1983;40:433–5.
2. Lee HB, Lyketsos CG. Delayed post-hypoxic leukoencephalopathy. Psychosomatics 2001;42:530–3.
3. Custodio CM, Basford JR. Delayed postanoxic encephalopathy: a case report and literature review. Arch Phys Med Rehabil 2004;85:502–5.
4. Plum F, Posner JB, Hain RF. Delayed neurological deterioration after anoxia. Arch Intern Med 1962;110:18–25.
5. Hori A, Hirose G, Kataoka S, et al. Delayed postanoxic encephalopathy after strangulation. Serial neuroradiological and neurochemical studies. Arch Neurol 1991;48:871–4.
6. Mizutani T, Shiozawa R, Takemori S, et al. Delayed post-anoxic encephalopathy without relation to carbon monoxide poisoning. Intern Med 1993;32:430–3.
7. Weinberger LM, Schmidley JW, Schafer IA, et al. Delayed postanoxic demyelination and arylsulfatase-A pseudodeficiency. Neurology 1994;44:152–4.
8. Protass LM. Delayed postanoxic encephalopathy after heroin use. Ann Intern Med 1971;74:738–9.
9. Barnett MH, Miller LA, Reddel SW, et al. Reversible delayed leukoencephalopathy following intravenous heroin overdose. J Clin Neurosci 2001;8:165–7.
10. Shprecher D, Mehta L. The syndrome of delayed post-hypoxic leukoencephalopathy. NeuroRehabilitation 2010;26:65–72.
11. Lee MS, Marsden CD. Neurological sequelae following carbon monoxide poisoning clinical course and outcome according to the clinical types and brain computed tomography scan findings. Mov Disord 1994;9:550–8.
12. Chen-Plotkin AS, Pau KT, Schmahmann JD. Delayed leukoencephalopathy after hypoxic-ischemic injury. Arch Neurol 2008;65:144–5.
13. Gottfried JA, Mayer SA, Shungu DC, et al. Delayed posthypoxic demyelination. Association with arylsulfatase A deficiency and lactic acidosis on proton MR spectroscopy. Neurology 1997;49:1400–4.
14. Posner JB, Saper CB, Schiff ND, et al. Plum and Posner's diagnosis of stupor and coma. 4th edition. New York: Oxford University Press; 2007. p. 210–1.
15. Heckmann JG, Erbguth F, Neundörfer B. Delayed postanoxic demyelination registry. Neurology 1998;51:1235–6.
16. Shprecher DR, Flanigan KM, Smith AG, et al. Clinical and diagnostic features of delayed hypoxic leukoencephalopathy. J Neuropsychiatry Clin Neurosci 2008;20:473–7.
17. Khot S, Walker M, Lacy JM, et al. An unsuccessful trial of immunomodulatory therapy in delayed posthypoxic demyelination. Neurocrit Care 2007;7:253–6.
18. Molloy S, Soh C, Williams TL. Reversible delayed posthypoxic leukoencephalopathy. AJNR Am J Neuroradiol 2006;27:1763–5.
19. Min SK. A brain syndrome associated with delayed neuropsychiatric sequelae following acute carbon monoxide intoxication. Acta Psychiatr Scand 1986;73:80–6.
20. Kawada N, Ochiai N, Kuzuhara S. Diffusion MRI in acute carbon monoxide poisoning. Intern Med 2004;43:639–40.

21. Singhal AB, Topcuoglu MA, Koroshetz WJ. Diffusion MRI in three types of anoxic encephalopathy. J Neurol Sci 2002;196:37–40.
22. Choi IS, Lee MS, Lee YJ, et al. Technetium-99m HM-PAO SPECT in patients with delayed neurologic sequelae after carbon monoxide poisoning. J Korean Med Sci 1992;7:11–8.
23. Choi IS, Kim SK, Lee SS, et al. Evaluation of outcome of delayed neurologic sequelae after carbon monoxide poisoning by technetium-99m hexamethylpropylene amine oxime brain single photon emission computed tomography. Eur Neurol 1995;35:137–42.
24. Norkool DM, Kirkpatrick JN. Treatment of acute carbon monoxide poisoning with hyperbaric oxygen: a review of 115 cases. Ann Emerg Med 1985;14:1168–71.
25. Myers RA. Carbon monoxide poisoning. J Emerg Med 1984;1:245–8.
26. Kao LW, Nañagas KA. Carbon monoxide poisoning. Emerg Med Clin North Am 2004;22:985–1018.
27. Thom SR, Bhopale VM, Han ST, et al. Intravascular neutrophil activation due to carbon monoxide poisoning. Am J Respir Crit Care Med 2006;174:1239–48.
28. Raphael JC, Elkharrat D, Jars-Guincestre MC, et al. Trial of normobaric and hyperbaric oxygen for acute carbon monoxide intoxication. Lancet 1989;2:414–9.
29. Ducassé JL, Celsis P, Marc-Vergnes JP. Non-comatose patients with acute carbon monoxide poisoning: hyperbaric or normobaric oxygenation? Undersea Hyperb Med 1995;22:9–15.
30. Thom SR, Taber RL, Mendiguren II, et al. Delayed neuropsychologic sequelae after carbon monoxide poisoning: prevention by treatment with hyperbaric oxygen. Ann Emerg Med 1995;25:474–80.
31. Mathieu D, Wattel F, Mathieu-Nolf M, et al. Randomized prospective study comparing the effect of HBO versus 12 hours NBO in non-comatose CO poisoned patients: results of interim analysis [abstract]. Undersea Hyperb Med 1996;23:7–8.
32. Scheinkestel CD, Bailey M, Myles PS, et al. Hyperbaric or normobaric oxygen for acute carbon monoxide poisoning: a randomised controlled clinical trial. Med J Aust 1999;170:203–10.
33. Weaver LK, Hopkins RO, Chan KJ, et al. Hyperbaric oxygen for acute carbon monoxide poisoning. N Engl J Med 2002;347:1057–67.
34. Annane D, Chadda K, Gajdos P, et al. Hyperbaric oxygen therapy for acute domestic carbon monoxide poisoning: two randomized controlled trials. Intensive Care Med 2011;37:486–92.
35. Hampson NB, Mathieu D, Piantadosi CA, et al. Carbon monoxide poisoning: interpretation of randomized clinical trials and unresolved treatment issues. Undersea Hyperb Med 2001;28:157–64.
36. Strang J, Griffiths P, Gossop M. Heroin smoking by 'chasing the dragon': origins and history. Addiction 1997;92:673–83 [discussion: 685–95].
37. Hendriks VM, van den Brink W, Blanken P, et al. Heroin self-administration by means of 'chasing the dragon': pharmacodynamics and bioavailability of inhaled heroin. Eur Neuropsychopharmacol 2001;11:241–52.
38. Wolters EC, van Wijngaarden GK, Stam FC, et al. Leucoencephalopathy after inhaling "heroin" pyrolysate. Lancet 1982;2:1233–7.
39. Offiah C, Hall E. Heroin-induced leukoencephalopathy: characterization using MRI, diffusion-weighted imaging, and MR spectroscopy. Clin Radiol 2008;63:146–52.
40. Long H, Deore K, Hoffman RS, et al. A fatal case of spongiform leukoencephalopathy linked to "chasing the dragon". J Toxicol Clin Toxicol 2003;41:887–91.

41. Kriegstein AR, Shungu DC, Millar WS, et al. Leukoencephalopathy and raised brain lactate from heroin vapor inhalation ("chasing the dragon"). Neurology 1999;53:1765–73.
42. Buxton JA, Sebastian R, Clearsky L, et al. Chasing the dragon- Characterizing cases of leukoencephalopathy associated with heroin inhalation in British Columbia. Harm Reduct J 2011;8:3.
43. Weber W, Henkes H, Möller P, et al. Toxic spongiform leucoencephalopathy after inhaling heroin vapour. Eur Radiol 1998;8:749–55.
44. Kriegstein AR, Armitage BA, Kim PY. Heroin inhalation and progressive spongiform leukoencephalopathy. N Engl J Med 1997;336:589–90.
45. Gupta PK, Krishnan PR, Sudhakar PJ. Hippocampal involvement due to heroin inhalation–"chasing the dragon". Clin Neurol Neurosurg 2009;111:278–81.
46. Tan TP, Algra PR, Valk J, et al. Toxic leukoencephalopathy after inhalation of poisoned heroin: MR findings. AJNR Am J Neuroradiol 1994;15:175–8.
47. Celius EG, Andersson S. Leucoencephalopathy after inhalation of heroin: a case report. J Neurol Neurosurg Psychiatry 1996;60:694–5.
48. Gacouin A, Lavoue S, Signouret T, et al. Reversible spongiform leucoencephalopathy after inhalation of heated heroin. Intensive Care Med 2003;29:1012–5.
49. Keogh CF, Andrews GT, Spacey SD, et al. Neuroimaging features of heroin inhalation toxicity: "chasing the dragon". AJR Am J Roentgenol 2003;180:847–50.
50. Hagel J, Andrews G, Vertinsky T, et al. "Chasing the dragon"—imaging of heroin inhalation leukoencephalopathy. Can Assoc Radiol J 2005;56:199–203.
51. Bartlett E, Mikulis DJ. Chasing "chasing the dragon" with MRI: leukoencephalopathy in drug abuse. Br J Radiol 2005;78:997–1004.
52. Au-Yeung K, Lai C. Toxic leucoencephalopathy after heroin inhalation. Australas Radiol 2002;46:306–8.
53. Ryan A, Molloy FM, Farrell MA, et al. Fatal toxic leukoencephalopathy: clinical, radiological, and necropsy findings in two patients. J Neurol Neurosurg Psychiatry 2005;76:1014–6.
54. Chen CY, Lee KW, Lee CC, et al. Heroin-induced spongiform leukoencephalopathy: value of diffusion MR imaging. J Comput Assist Tomogr 2000;24:735–7.
55. Maschke M, Fehlings T, Kastrup O, et al. Toxic leukoencephalopathy after intravenous consumption of heroin and cocaine with unexpected clinical recovery. J Neurol 1999;246:850–1.
56. Chang WC, Lo CP, Kao HW, et al. MRI features of spongiform leukoencephalopathy following heroin inhalation. Neurology 2006;67:504.
57. Brenneisen R, Hasler F. GC/MS determination of pyrolysis products from diacetylmorphine and adulterants of street heroin samples. J Forensic Sci 2002;47:885–8.
58. Sempere AP, Posada I, Ramo C, et al. Spongiform leucoencephalopathy after inhaling heroin. Lancet 1991;338:320.
59. Büttner A, Mall G, Penning R, et al. The neuropathology of heroin abuse. Forensic Sci Int 2000;113:435–42.
60. Halloran O, Ifthikharuddin S, Samkoff L. Leukoencephalopathy from "chasing the dragon". Neurology 2005;64:1755.
61. Hinchey J, Chaves C, Appignani B, et al. A reversible posterior leukoencephalopathy syndrome. N Engl J Med 1996;334:494–500.
62. Bartynski WS. Posterior reversible encephalopathy syndrome, part 1: fundamental imaging and clinical features. AJNR Am J Neuroradiol 2008;29:1036–42.
63. Mukherjee P, McKinstry RC. Reversible posterior leukoencephalopathy syndrome: evaluation with diffusion-tensor MR imaging. Radiology 2001;219:756–65.

64. Glusker P, Recht L, Lane B. Reversible posterior leukoencephalopathy syndrome and bevacizumab. N Engl J Med 2006;354:980–2 [discussion: 980–2].
65. Incecik F, Hergüner MO, Altunbasak S, et al. Evaluation of nine children with reversible posterior encephalopathy syndrome. Neurol India 2009;57:475–8.
66. Dicuonzo F, Salvati A, Palma M, et al. Posterior reversible encephalopathy syndrome associated with methotrexate neurotoxicity: conventional magnetic resonance and diffusion-weighted imaging findings. J Child Neurol 2009;24: 1013–8.
67. Mavragani CP, Vlachoyiannopoulos PG, Kosmas N, et al. A case of reversible posterior leucoencephalopathy syndrome after rituximab infusion. Rheumatology 2004;43:1450–1.
68. Moskowitz A, Nolan C, Lis E, et al. Posterior reversible encephalopathy syndrome due to sirolimus. Bone Marrow Transplant 2007;39:653–4.
69. Govindarajan R, Adusumilli J, Baxter DL, et al. Reversible posterior leukoencephalopathy syndrome induced by RAF kinase inhibitor BAY 43-9006. J Clin Oncol 2006;24:e48.
70. Cumurciuc R, Martinez-Almoyna L, Henry C, et al. Posterior reversible encephalopathy syndrome during sunitinib therapy. Rev Neurol (Paris) 2008;164:605–7.
71. Kappos L, Antel J, Comi G, et al. Oral fingolimod (FTY720) for relapsing multiple sclerosis. N Engl J Med 2006;355:1124–40.
72. Koichihara R, Hamano SI, Yamashita S, et al. Posterior reversible encephalopathy syndrome associated with IVIG in a patient with Guillain-Barré syndrome. Pediatr Neurol 2008;39:123–5.
73. Belmouaz S, Desport E, Leroy F, et al. Posterior reversible encephalopathy induced by intravenous immunoglobulin. Nephrol Dial Transplant 2008;23:417–9.
74. De Klippel N, Sennesael J, Lamote J, et al. Cyclosporin leukoencephalopathy induced by intravenous lipid solution. Lancet 1992;339:1114.
75. Wu Q, Marescaux C, Wolff V, et al. Tacrolimus-associated posterior reversible encephalopathy syndrome after solid organ transplantation. Eur Neurol 2010; 64:169–77.
76. Bodkin CL, Eidelman BH. Sirolimus-induced posterior reversible encephalopathy. Neurology 2007;68:2039–40.
77. Ito Y, Arahata Y, Goto Y, et al. Cisplatin neurotoxicity presenting as reversible posterior leukoencephalopathy syndrome. AJNR Am J Neuroradiol 1998;19:415–7.
78. Hommaway C, Mian A, Nagy Z. Images in haematology. Irreversible blindness secondary to posterior reversible encephalopathy syndrome following CHOP combination chemotherapy. Br J Haematol 2010;150:129.
79. Russell MT, Nassif AS, Cacayorin ED, et al. Gemcitabine-associated posterior reversible encephalopathy syndrome: MR imaging and MR spectroscopy findings. Magn Reson Imaging 2001;19:129–32.
80. Tam CS, Galanos J, Seymour JF, et al. Reversible posterior leukoencephalopathy syndrome complicating cytotoxic chemotherapy for hematologic malignancies. Am J Hematol 2004;77:72–6.
81. Reece DE, Frei-Lahr DA, Shepherd JD, et al. Neurologic complications in allogeneic bone marrow transplant patients receiving cyclosporin. Bone Marrow Transplant 1991;8:393–401.
82. Vaughn DJ, Jarvik JG, Hackney D, et al. High-dose cytarabine neurotoxicity: MR findings during the acute phase. AJNR Am J Neuroradiol 1993;14:1014–6.
83. Bartynski WS, Zeigler Z, Spearman MP, et al. Etiology of cortical and white matter lesions in cyclosporin-A and FK-506 neurotoxicity. AJNR Am J Neuroradiol 2001;22:1901–14.

84. Mahoney DH Jr, Shuster JJ, Nitschke R, et al. Acute neurotoxicity in children with B-precursor acute lymphoid leukemia: an association with intermediate-dose intravenous methotrexate and intrathecal triple therapy–a Pediatric Oncology Group study. J Clin Oncol 1998;16:1712–22.
85. Asato R, Akiyama Y, Ito M, et al. Nuclear magnetic resonance abnormalities of the cerebral white matter in children with acute lymphoblastic leukemia and malignant lymphoma during and after central nervous system prophylactic treatment with intrathecal methotrexate. Cancer 1992;70:1997–2004.
86. Bartynski WS, Tan HP, Boardman JF, et al. Posterior reversible encephalopathy syndrome after solid organ transplantation. AJNR Am J Neuroradiol 2008;29: 924–30.
87. Wong R, Beguelin GZ, de Lima M, et al. Tacrolimus-associated posterior reversible encephalopathy syndrome after allogeneic haematopoietic stem cell transplantation. Br J Haematol 2003;122:128–34.
88. Noè A, Cappelli B, Biffi A, et al. High incidence of severe cyclosporine neurotoxicity in children affected by haemoglobinopaties undergoing myeloablative haematopoietic stem cell transplantation: early diagnosis and prompt intervention ameliorates neurological outcome. Ital J Pediatr 2010;36:14.
89. Duncan R, Hadley D, Bone I, et al. Blindness in eclampsia: CT and MR imaging. J Neurol Neurosurg Psychiatry 1989;52:899–902.
90. Schwartz RB, Jones KM, Kalina P, et al. Hypertensive encephalopathy: findings on CT, MR imaging, and SPECT imaging in 14 cases. AJR Am J Roentgenol 1992;159:379–83.
91. McKinney AM, Short J, Truwit CL, et al. Posterior reversible encephalopathy syndrome: incidence of atypical regions of involvement and imaging findings. AJR Am J Roentgenol 2007;189:904–12.
92. Donmez FY, Basaran C, Kayahan Ulu EM, et al. MRI features of posterior reversible encephalopathy syndrome in 33 patients. J Neuroimaging 2010;20:22–8.
93. Finocchi V, Bozzao A, Bonamini M, et al. Magnetic resonance imaging in posterior reversible encephalopathy syndrome: report of three cases and review of literature. Arch Gynecol Obstet 2005;271:79–85.
94. Casey SO, Sampaio RC, Michel E, et al. Posterior reversible encephalopathy syndrome: utility of fluid-attenuated inversion recovery MR imaging in the detection of cortical and subcortical lesions. AJNR Am J Neuroradiol 2000;21:1199–206.
95. Ay H, Buonanno FS, Schaefer PW, et al. Posterior leukoencephalopathy without severe hypertension: utility of diffusion-weighted MRI. Neurology 1998;51: 1369–76.
96. Henderson RD, Rajah T, Nicol AJ, et al. Posterior leukoencephalopathy following intrathecal chemotherapy with MRA-documented vasospasm. Neurology 2003; 60:326–8.
97. Thaipisuttikul I, Phanthumchinda K. Recurrent reversible posterior leukoencephalopathy in a patient with systemic lupus erythematosus. J Neurol 2005; 252:230–1.
98. Sweany JM, Bartynski WS, Boardman JF. "Recurrent" posterior reversible encephalopathy syndrome: report of 3 cases–PRES can strike twice! J Comput Assist Tomogr 2007;31:148–56.
99. Bartynski WS, Boardman JF. Catheter angiography, MR angiography, and MR perfusion in posterior reversible encephalopathy syndrome. AJNR Am J Neuroradiol 2008;29:447–55.
100. Ito T, Sakai T, Inagawa S, et al. MR angiography of cerebral vasospasm in preeclampsia. AJNR Am J Neuroradiol 1995;16:1344–6.

101. Lin JT, Wang SJ, Fuh JL, et al. Prolonged reversible vasospasm in cyclosporin A-induced encephalopathy. AJNR Am J Neuroradiol 2003;24:102–4.
102. Ito Y, Niwa H, Iida T, et al. Post-transfusion reversible posterior leukoencephalopathy syndrome with cerebral vasoconstriction. Neurology 1997;49:1174–5.
103. Trommer BL, Homer D, Mikhael MA. Cerebral vasospasm and eclampsia. Stroke 1988;19:326–9.
104. Bartynski WS, Sanghvi A. Neuroimaging of delayed eclampsia. Report of 3 cases and review of the literature. J Comput Assist Tomogr 2003;27:699–713.
105. Aeby A, David P, Fricx C, et al. Posterior reversible encephalopathy syndrome revealing acute post-streptococcal glomerulonephritis. J Child Neurol 2006; 21:250–1.
106. Geraghty JJ, Hoch DB, Robert ME, et al. Fatal puerperal cerebral vasospasm and stroke in a young woman. Neurology 1991;41:1145–7.
107. Apollon KM, Robinson JN, Schwartz RB, et al. Cortical blindness in severe preeclampsia: computed tomography, magnetic resonance imaging, and single-photon-emission computed tomography findings. Obstet Gynecol 2000; 95:1017–9.
108. Sanchez-Carpintero R, Narbona J, López de Mesa R, et al. Transient posterior encephalopathy induced by chemotherapy in children. Pediatr Neurol 2001; 24:145–8.
109. Naidu K, Moodley J, Corr P, et al. Single photon emission and cerebral computerised tomographic scan and transcranial Doppler sonographic findings in eclampsia. Br J Obstet Gynaecol 1997;104:1165–72.
110. Edvinsson L, Owman C, Sjöberg NO. Autonomic nerves, mast cells, and amine receptors in human brain vessels. A histochemical and pharmacological study. Brain Res 1976;115:377–93.
111. Beausang-Linder M, Bill A. Cerebral circulation in acute arterial hypertension—protective effects of sympathetic nervous activity. Acta Physiol Scand 1981;111: 193–9.
112. Bartynski WS. Posterior reversible encephalopathy syndrome, part 2: controversies surrounding pathophysiology of vasogenic edema. AJNR Am J Neuroradiol 2008;29:1043–9.
113. Lanzino G, Cloft H, Hemstreet MK, et al. Reversible posterior leukoencephalopathy following organ transplantation. Description of two cases. Clin Neurol Neurosurg 1997;99:222–6.
114. Thyagarajan GK, Cobanoglu A, Johnston W. FK506-induced fulminant leukoencephalopathy after single-lung transplantation. Ann Thorac Surg 1997;64(14): 61–4.
115. Schiff D, Lopes MB. Neuropathological correlates of reversible posterior leukoencephalopathy. Neurocrit Care 2005;2:303–5.
116. Greenwood MJ, Dodds AJ, Garricik R, et al. Posterior leukoencephalopathy in association with the tumour lysis syndrome in acute lymphoblastic leukaemia—a case with clinicopathological correlation. Leuk Lymphoma 2003;44:719–21.
117. Cain MS, Burton GV, Holcombe RF. Fatal leukoencephalopathy in a patient with non-Hodgkin's lymphoma treated with CHOP chemotherapy and high-dose steroids. Am J Med Sci 1998;315:202–7.

Heavy Metal Chelation in Neurotoxic Exposures

David H. Jang, MD*, Robert S. Hoffman, MD, FRCPEdin

KEYWORDS

- Heavy metals • Chelation • Postchelation challenge
- Neurotoxic

A common definition of a metal is an electropositive element that is a conductor of heat and electricity and typically forms a salt with a nonmetal. Although this includes transition metals such as iron and copper, it also includes lanthanides, actinides, and metalloids. Most living organisms require varying amounts of certain metals such as iron, copper, and zinc to survive. Some metals, such as aluminum, are considered nonessential and are classified as trace elements. Other metals such as cadmium, mercury, and lead have no known biologic role in humans and thus are toxic with sufficient accumulation. The term heavy metals is loosely applied to describe elements with a specific gravity greater than 5 times the density of water.[1] Many other definitions have been proposed for the term heavy metals. Some definitions are based on the density, atomic number/weight, or the potential to cause human toxicity affecting multiple organs such as the nervous system. Regardless of whether they have a biologic role in humans, all metals are capable of toxicity as dose increases.

The use of metals dates back thousands of years. For example, medicinal agents, such as colloidal silver, were prescribed for gonorrhea and the common cold. Nefarious purposes are also documented and intentional poisonings with arsenic and thallium still continue today.[2–7]

Metals are of public interest because of exposures related to environmental contamination and through bioaccumulation within the food chain. One of the most devastating complications of poisoning from environmental metal contamination occurred in the 1950s in Minamata Bay, a fishing community in Japan near a vinyl chloride plant. Methylmercury (organic mercury) accumulated in the marine life and resulted in mass poisoning; particularly devastating neurologic sequelae were seen in newborns, who are more susceptible than adults to neurotoxins. Another devastating environmental

Disclosures: The authors have nothing to disclose.
Department of Emergency Medicine, New York University School of Medicine, Bellevue Hospital Center, New York, NY, USA
* Corresponding author. 455 First Avenue, Room 123, New York, NY 10016.
E-mail address: jangd01@nyumc.org

Neurol Clin 29 (2011) 607–622
doi:10.1016/j.ncl.2011.05.002
0733-8619/11/$ – see front matter © 2011 Elsevier Inc. All rights reserved.

exposure occurred in Bangladesh, where likely millions of people were/are chronically exposed to low concentrations of arsenic in drinking water from wells dug into a contaminated aquifer.[8] Occupational exposure may also be a source of metal poisoning such as cadmium.[9]

Currently, metal poisoning is a subject of debate in many areas such as human development and general health. There is widespread concern regarding the safety of various sources of potential metal toxicity such as dental amalgams, metal alloy prosthesis, seafood, and even vaccines. Dental amalgams consisting of silver-mercury have been used for more than 100 years without any overt effects. Despite this, concern for mercury toxicity continues. In the 1970s it was found that amalgams can release mercury vapors in concentrations higher than what is deemed safe by accepted occupational guidelines. It was later realized that the volume of inhaled mercury vapors was small and, to date, there are no proven adverse effects associated with dental amalgams.[10] Another mercury concern comes from a popular belief that links mercury-containing thimerosal in vaccines with autism. Again, although there is no proven association, this belief continues.[11,12] The most recent concern about metal toxicity involves total joint replacements. This concern stems from the degradation of prosthetic joints with the release into the blood of various alloys such as chromium, titanium, and cobalt. Studies have measured increased blood concentrations of metals found in alloy prostheses, and case reports clearly suggest toxicity. Despite this, the overall risk of metal toxicity from prosthetic failure remains unquantified.[13–15]

Metals often exist in various forms that may have different toxicities. For example, arsenic is a metalloid that can exist in the elemental, inorganic, or organic form. Elemental arsenic is considered nontoxic because of its insolubility.[16] This is in contrast with inorganic arsenic salts, which include the pentavalent (arsenate) and trivalent (arsenite) forms, and which are associated with profound cardiac, gastrointestinal, neurologic, and hematologic toxicity. With metals such as antimony and arsenic, the trivalent form is considered more toxic than pentavalent compounds because of the higher affinity for erythrocytes and sulfhydryl groups.[17] Other examples where the form of the metal is an important determinate of toxicity are mercury and lead.

Many metals, for example mercury, have a high affinity for electron-donor ligands such as sulfhydryl groups. These metals can affect structural proteins, receptors, and enzyme systems. Others metals are chemically similar to cations that participate in enzymatic processes; for example, lead is chemically similar to calcium, which explains the multisystem impact that lead has on calcium-dependant systems such as second-messenger systems and apotosis.[18,19] Likewise, thallium and potassium have similar ionic radii and, as a result, thallium accumulates in the nervous system and cardiovascular system as if it were potassium.[20,21] The central nervous system is often a target of numerous metals because of their multisystem effects. Metals such as lead, manganese, mercury, and thallium are well known for their toxicity on the nervous system, particularly the alkyl derivatives of metals such as lead and mercury. Many of these metals cause neurotoxicity by interfering with neurotransmitters and membrane transport or by binding with cations such as calcium.

CLINICAL FEATURES

The toxic clinical manifestations of metal poisoning depend on several factors that include, but are not limited to the amount and form of the metal, the chronicity of the ingestion, the route of exposure, and the general health of the individual.[22]

Acute metal poisoning results from a large exposure in a short period of time, whereas chronic metal poisoning results from low-dose exposures, typically from environmental and occupational sources, in a longer period of time. Because the clinical presentation of chronic poisoning can differ from acute poisoning, it is crucial that clinicians remain aware of these differences when considering diagnosis and treatment options.

Acute metal poisoning is typically a multiorgan disorder commonly involving the gastrointestinal, central nervous and peripheral nervous system, kidney, and hair and nails. As a general rule, an acute oral ingestion of a significant amount of metal salts causes gastrointestinal symptoms such as nausea, emesis, abdominal pain, and diarrhea. Cardiovascular manifestations ranging from sinus tachycardia and orthostatic hypotension to lethal dysrhythmias can occur following acute ingestion. Acute encephalopathy can also develop and progress for several days, which may manifest as seizures, delirium, or coma. A metallic taste or oropharyngeal irritation may occur. In many instances, other organ systems, such as the pulmonary and endocrine systems, are also affected. **Table 1** lists the major clinical findings for many metal exposures. In contrast, chronic metal poisoning is subtler and often includes dermatologic and peripheral nervous system findings.

The nervous system serves as one of the toxic targets of many metals, and this may occur for numerous reasons such as mimicking common cations used as messengers; for example, thallium can mimic potassium and lead can mimic calcium.[5,6,22] Metals in the nervous system may also inhibit various enzymes, disrupt membranes, and damage structural proteins. Some metals, such as manganese, manifest primarily as neuropsychiatric problems. Manganese toxicity is often described as biphasic. This toxicity includes the acute phase, which includes behavioral changes and anxiety, and the second phase, which manifests as late-developing movement disorders such as tremor, ataxia, and loss of facial expression. These extrapyramidal movements are similar to those seen Parkinson disease except they are often accompanied by only mild cognitive involvement and are less likely to respond to levodopa.[23,24]

Some metals may cause encephalopathy. Patients with acute aluminum toxicity may develop myoclonic encephalopathy and seizures within days to weeks after a substantial systemic aluminum exposure. Chronic aluminum toxicity causes a microcytic hypochromic anemia along with osteomalacia and dementia. The primary neurologic disturbances found with chronic aluminum toxicity are speech disturbance, myoclonic jerks, EEG abnormalities, and dementia; these symptoms are often termed dialysis dementia because initial reports involved patients on dialysis who underwent hemodialysis with fluids contaminated with aluminum.[25,26] Chronic bismuth toxicity is associated with a diffuse progressive encephalopathy that may start as irritability but, with continued exposure, progresses to myoclonus, ataxia, and coma, followed by death in severe cases.[27,28]

Other metal exposures may result in peripheral nervous system findings. For instance, arsenic may cause a peripheral neuropathy 1 to 3 weeks after exposure. Often, sensory neuropathies develop in a stocking-glove distribution manifesting as tingling and numbness along with diminished sensation to temperature and pain. In severe cases, a motor neuropathy may develop that includes weakness or ascending paralysis similar to Guillain-Barré syndrome.[29,30] Thallium poisoning is another example of a metal that may result in both central and peripheral nervous system findings. Neurologic symptoms usually appear 2 to 5 days following an acute exposure. Although confusion, seizures, and ataxia are common, perhaps the most characteristic finding of thallium toxicity is a severely painful ascending peripheral neuropathy that rapidly progresses.[31]

Table 1
Major clinical features of metal poisoning

Metal	Acute Poisoning	Chronic Poisoning
Antimony	Mucosal irritation and ulcers, hemorrhagic gastritis, acute lung injury, QT prolongation, nausea, vomiting and diarrhea	Papules and pustules around sebaceous/sweat glands (antimony spots), pancytopenia
Arsenic	Nausea, vomiting, cholera-like diarrhea, acute lung injury, QT prolongation, tachycardia/hypotension, torsades de pointes	Encephalopathy, cerebral edema, peripheral neuropathy (sensory>motor), hepatic angiosarcoma, aplasia, alopecia, diffuse pruritic macular rash, Mees lines
Bismuth	Acute renal failure, abdominal pain	Myoclonic encephalopathy (can mimic Creutzfeldt-Jacob disease), blue-black discoloration of gums (bismuth lines)
Cadmium	Nausea, vomiting, and diarrhea	Link to parkinsonism, olfactory disturbances, restrictive lung disease, pulmonary fibrosis, acute renal failure, osteomalacia (itai-itai disease)
Chromium	Nausea, vomiting, and diarrhea; hemolysis; disseminated intravascular coagulation, corrosive burns (Cr^{6+}), contact dermatitis (Cr^{3+})	Nasal septal perforation, pulmonary fibrosis, pneumoconiosis, occupational asthma
Cobalt	Cardiomyopathy, polycythemia, thyroid/goiter/hyperplasia	Cardiomyopathy, asthma, polycythemia, dermatitis, decreased proprioception, altered CN VIII function, visual and hearing problems (in prosthetic joints)
Copper	Nausea, vomiting, and diarrhea (bluish color); conjunctiva irritation; hypotension; hemolysis	Hepatolenticular degeneration, hepatotoxicity, Kayser-Fleischer rings

Lead	Acute encephalopathy, abdominal pain, constipation	Peripheral neuropathy (motor, arms>legs), developmental delay, cognitive problems, hypertension, nephropathy (Fanconi syndrome)
Manganese	Psychiatric (manganese madness)	Psychiatric (manganese madness), parkinsonism, reactive airway disease
Mercury[a]	Nausea, vomiting, and diarrhea; pneumonitis (elemental); renal dysfunction	Choreoathetosis and spasmodic ballismus, neurasthenia and erethism, renal dysfunction, acrodynia (pink disease), cerebellar dysfunction, constricted visual fields (organic)
Nickel[b]	Cerebral edema, acute lung injury	Interstitial pneumonitis, myocarditis, nickel dermatitis
Selenium[c]	Gastrointestinal mucosal injury, conjunctiva edema, reversible anosmia	Brittle hair/pruritic scalp rash, brittle nails with red/white ridges, hyperreflexia, peripheral paresthesia
Silver	None	Skin discoloration from ingesting colloidal silver (argyria)
Thallium[d]	Altered mental status, painful ascending neuropathy (sensory>motor), optic neuropathy, autonomic neuropathy, hypertension, abdominal pain, nausea, vomiting, constipation	Alopecia, Mees lines
Zinc[e]	Nausea, vomiting, and diarrhea; transient anosmia; metal fume fever (welding); abdominal pain	Sideroblastic anemia, myelodysplastic syndrome, anemia and granulocytopenia, linked with multiple sclerosis, myeloneuropathy (from copper deficiency)

[a] Organic mercury causes neurologic dysfunction that can be delayed in onset and is largely irreversible.
[b] Organic nickel (nickel carbonyl) is the most important source of nondermatologic toxicity.
[c] Most toxicity associated with selenious acid compounds.
[d] Alopecia and peripheral neuropathy are characteristic findings.
[e] Most toxicity associated with zinc salts (eg, zinc chloride).

DIAGNOSTIC TESTING

The diagnosis of metal poisoning relies primarily on clinical history and physical findings combined with proper laboratory testing. It is important to determine whether the exposure is acute, subacute, or chronic because this affects the timing and interpretation of test results. Confounding factors that may result in misinterpretation of test results should also be considered. An example of a common confounder occurs in the evaluation of possible arsenic poisoning. Failure to consider food-derived organic arsenicals when obtaining a urinary arsenic concentration can result in an erroneous assumption of arsenic poisoning.[32] This may result in harm to the patient, both by failing to identify the true cause of their symptoms but also by exposing them to unnecessary, expensive, and potentially harmful treatment.[33]

Acute metal salt toxicity often results in volume depletion and kidney injury so standard laboratory testing including a complete blood count, electrolytes, renal function, and a urinalysis should be obtained. More specific testing may be required depending on the exposure. An example is testing for bilirubin and haptoglobin, markers of hemolysis, after copper exposure.[34] An electrocardiogram should be obtained to evaluate for dysrhythmias and QT prolongation, which can occur with antimony and arsenic toxicity.[35–37]

Although metal toxicity can be suspected based on clinical presentation and standard laboratory testing alone, in many cases the diagnosis relies on obtaining a specific metal concentration in blood or a 24-hour urine collection. When obtaining a 24-hour urine collection, it is important to understand the variation in the urinary excretion of both organic substances and metals during a normal day. The most common method to correct for this involves the calculation of the urinary metal/creatinine concentration ratios. This calculation assumes that the daily creatinine excretion rate is stable and helps to account for variation in urinary flow.[38,39] A serum metal concentration can also be obtained, which, along with speciation, can determine the valance state of the metal. However, speciation may be difficult to obtain depending on the metal. For example, differentiation between Cr^{3+} and Cr^{6+} is difficult, so instead a total chromium concentration is reported. In acute life-threatening metal toxicity, a spot urine metal concentration may be sent before the initiation of chelation therapy. Although an increased spot urine test is confirmatory in a patient with a characteristic clinical presentation of acute metal toxicity, a normal concentration does not entirely exclude the diagnosis.[40] A study of 9 patients with acute arsenic toxicity shows the wide range in spot urine arsenic concentrations, which ranged from 192 to 198,450 µg/L.[41] Definitive diagnosis often relies on a proper 24-hour urine collection. Testing for suspected metal poisoning should be based on clinical presentation as opposed to a shotgun approach of obtaining a metal panel that may only confuse the evaluation with marginally abnormal values. Another important consideration is that samples should be sent to an accredited laboratory with experience in the measurement of metals.[42]

Radiographic imaging can be diagnostic in the appropriate clinical context. An abdominal radiograph is often obtained to evaluate for possible acute metal ingestion. An ingestion of a metal such as lead may result in radiopaque opacities within the gastrointestinal tract. However, neither the sensitivity nor the specificity of radiographs is well established. Thus, although a positive finding is highly suggestive, a negative abdominal radiograph should not be used to exclude a potential toxic metal ingestion.[43] A chest radiograph should be obtained in patients who present with pulmonary complaints such as dyspnea and chest pain; acute exposures to certain metal fumes, such as cadmium or mercury, can result in delayed and progressive acute lung injury leading to death.[44]

Many metal exposures manifest with only neurologic symptoms, which can range from the exquisitely painful neuropathy of acute thallium exposure to myoclonic encephalopathy from chronic bismuth exposure.[27,45,46] Nerve conduction studies can be used to diagnose an axonopathy, the most common form of peripheral nervous system disease. Nerve conduction studies measure both the motor compound action potential as well as sensory nerve action potential. A measure of the sensory nerve action potential is considered a more sensitive test than motor compound action potential. A nerve biopsy can also be performed to confirm degeneration of both the myelin sheath and axons, although the findings depend on where the biopsy is performed. For example, in the case of arsenic-related peripheral neuropathy, axonal loss begins in the distal lower extremities so a biopsy in this area would likely result in a higher yield.[47,48] Other tests, such as positron emission tomography studies, have also been used in the case of suspected manganese toxicity. Magnetic resonance imaging (MRI) abnormalities can also be seen with manganese-associated parkinsonism, which often shows abnormal T1-weighted signal hyperintensity in the basal ganglia, particularly in the globus pallidus with normal T2-weighted images.[49,50] The results of these tests are not specific for metal poisoning and can occur in other neurologic disorders, so results should be applied in the correct clinical context.

Certain metals accumulate in specific compartments of the body, which may also aid in the diagnosis of metal poisoning. Lead accumulates in the teeth (particularly the dentine of children). It also can interfere with normal calcium deposition in developing bones (especially the growth plates), which can manifest as lead lines; this finding may help assess lead exposure in young children.[51] Analysis of hair and nails is also sometimes used to aid in the diagnosis of certain metal poisonings such as arsenic, mercury, and thallium. Arsenic can be detected in the proximal roots of hair in as little as 30 hours after an acute exposure.[52] However, the use of hair analysis for mercury poisoning is not recommended because hair avidly binds mercury from the environment, which makes this method unreliable.[53] Although the use of hair and nail analysis can be useful adjunctive testing, the use of blood and urine testing is highly recommended.

POSTCHELATION CHALLENGE URINARY METAL TESTING

Postchelation challenge testing grew out of a clinical decision rule developed for lead testing that was known as the calcium disodium edetate (CaNa$_2$EDTA) challenge test. The test was designed to determine whether asymptomatic patients with mildly increased blood concentrations of lead (25–35 μg/dL) were candidates for a full course of chelation therapy.[54–57] Patients who were symptomatic or had a significantly increased blood lead concentrations underwent full chelation without a provocation challenge. The challenge test was performed as follows: patients with increased blood concentrations of lead, in the 25 to 35 μg/dL range, were given a test dose of CaNa$_2$EDTA followed by a 24-hour urine lead collection. A ratio of the lead concentration in the urine to the dose of EDTA given is determined. A ratio of 0.7 or greater was considered positive and patients often underwent full chelation therapy. A ratio of 0.6 or less was negative and patients did not undergo chelation therapy.

Many variations in provocation testing have been described that used different chelation agents and shorter periods of urine collection to obtain a lead concentration. Shortened urinary lead collections were standardized in children but their use in adults has been questioned because of differences in kinetics of storage and variation in renal function compared with children.[58] A study that challenged this notion found that a 3-hour and 6-hour urine collection for lead concentration correlated well with the gold-standard 24-hour collection even in subjects with mild renal insufficiency.[59] Variations on the CaNa$_2$EDTA challenge were explored, such as a short-term course of alternating British antilewisite (BAL)-EDTA for the diagnostic testing of lead mobilization, which some believed would unmask a high lead burden more readily than the use of EDTA alone.[60]

Although the practice of provocation testing was common until the late 1960s, it was ultimately abandoned because of a lack of evidence for its usefulness as a diagnostic tool. In addition, experimental evidence showed the potential for harm caused by possible redistribution of lead from harmless body regions (eg, bone and muscle) into the brain of animals and from enhanced absorption of lead from the gastrointestinal tract.[61–63]

Urinary metal testing after chelation is used for a variety of reasons, such as in a patient who is acutely poisoned with a suspected metal where it may guide the decision to initiate chelation therapy. Urinary metal testing is also commonly used in the workplace to monitor exposure to certain metals, such as cadmium.[64] This testing is valid as long as it is applied in the appropriate clinical setting. An example would be a patient who presents with mood swings, ataxia, and renal insufficiency. A targeted urinary test for mercury would be appropriate in this clinical context. We recommend avoiding the use of a shotgun approach in ordering an entire metal screen panel because this only results in confusion and inappropriate treatment. The collection method, as well as analytical techniques, needs to be considered when interpreting the results of urinary metal test.[65] For example, prolonged storage of urine for arsenic testing can affect total arsenic recovery.

The timing of when a urine sample is obtained after a chelation agent is given may also result in misinterpretation. Urine samples collected in close proximity to the administration of chelation agents often result in increased concentrations of various metals, even metals such as zinc that are essential for normal health and function. Chelation agents commonly used in clinical practice, such as dimercaprol (BAL) and CaNa$_2$EDTA, bind and enhance elimination of various metals. Because metals of medical concern are found in the Earth's crust and our food chain, they are expected to be found in small amounts in urine and blood in both the healthy general population and those ill patients with disorders not related to metal poisoning.[66] The challenge is in distinguishing nonpoisoned patients with metal concentrations increased to more than the population norms from those who are poisoned.

To make the situation worse, urine metal concentrations may wrongly seem to be increased with chelators such as CaNa$_2$EDTA or succimer. In a study of 10 healthy individuals, a 24-hour urine collection was obtained with and without infusion of EDTA. The ratio of the increase of urinary elimination induced by EDTA was about double for iron and 5 times for aluminum and lead. Other studies confirm enhanced elimination of metals in nonpoisoned healthy volunteers given chelating agents with no bearing on toxicity.[66–69]

Similarly, asymptomatic workers exposed to mercury were challenged with dimercaptosuccinic acid (DMSA) as a measure of body burden. The average 24-hour mercury excretion was 4.3 μg/g of creatinine before chelation and 7.8 μg/g of creatinine after chelation.[70] Because most of the early excretion takes place after a chelation challenge, a provoked urine metal concentration may be even higher if the urine is collected in a shorter time period.

Proponents of provocative chelation testing argue that a reason for postchelation testing is to detect hidden body burdens of metals such as mercury and lead. The studies discussed earlier show that chelation provocative testing temporarily increases urine metal concentrations without any association with clinical toxicity. Practitioners of postprovocation testing compare increased postprovocation results with population norms, derived from nonprovoked specimens. Based on the false premise that reducing metal body burdens can ameliorate chronic symptoms of many diseases, such as autism, these practitioners use the results of provocative testing to initiate chelation, often at exorbitant fees.

An argument against the use of provocation testing is that most people are exposed to metals, mostly from bioaccumulation, without causing any toxicity. In a study of 17 children diagnosed with autism, a baseline 24-hour urine metal collection followed by a DMSA challenge, and repeat 24-hour urine metal analysis, showed that, when proper reference values were used and samples were adjusted for contamination such as a seafood diet, DMSA provocation did not result in excess chelatable burden of examined metals (arsenic, lead, and mercury).[71] However, these controls are rarely applied in practice, resulting in misinterpretation and unnecessary and potentially harmful treatment.

There are no normal values for provoked urine metal results in healthy asymptomatic individuals. Many smaller laboratories often use a lower reference value for unchallenged specimens typically used by major national laboratories. For example, smaller laboratories may use reference values of 3 $\mu g/g$ for mercury or 5 $\mu g/g$ for lead as a normal value, which is much lower than what is used by national laboratories (5 $\mu g/g$ for mercury or 150 $\mu g/g$ for lead).[72] Based on the use of these normal values, patients and their physicians are more likely to get abnormal results, which may initiate unnecessary evaluations and/or treatment that may cause both harm and financial loss to the patient. Practitioners who use provocative testing may use these results to have the patient undergo so-called detoxification with herbs, supplements, or intravenous chelation agents, which has resulted in deaths in inappropriately treated patients.[33,73]

In summary, the practice of postchelation urinary metal testing has no evidence to support its use and may result in potential harm to patients with no proven benefit. Even mildly increased concentrations of metals, especially with occupational exposure, often require just removal of the exposure. Chelation therapy is rarely required, especially if the patient has no symptoms. The American College of Medical Toxicology (ACMT) has released a position statement recommending against "the use of post-challenge urinary metal testing in clinical practice and the use of such test results as an indication for further administration of chelating agents."[74] This is in sharp contrast with patients who may present with symptoms of acute metal poisoning where there is a role for chelation therapy, as well as select patients who present with chronic metal toxicity based on a careful history and physical.

MANAGEMENT
General

Both acute and chronic metal poisoning can be life threatening and mandate early identification and aggressive treatment. Advanced life support such as endotracheal intubation should be initiated when necessary. Many patients with acute metal poisoning have decreased volume status from a combination of gastrointestinal losses and insensible losses. Careful attention to fluid balance is crucial, especially if there is any concern about concomitant cardiac dysfunction.

Gastrointestinal decontamination is often the next management decision considered once the patient has been stabilized. Many metals, such as iron, are often considered to poorly absorb to activated charcoal. However, activated charcoal has substantial binding to toxic metals such as mercury and thallium.[75–77] Given that small amounts of these metals may cause life-threatening toxicity, binding of even minute amounts of these metals may alter a patient's course, so activated charcoal should be administered after an acute exposure. Some metals, such as antimony, have also been shown to undergo enterohepatic circulation such that multiple-dose activated charcoal may also be of some benefit.[78]

If radiopaque material is shown in the gastrointestinal tract with a radiograph, whole-bowel irrigation with polyethylene glycol electrolyte lavage solution (PEG-ELS) should be initiated until there is clear effluent and the radiopaque material is no longer visualized on repeat radiograph.

Chelation Therapy

An important limitation in the discussion of chelators is the lack of large randomized controlled trials that show their efficacy. Most of the evidence in support of chelating agents is derived from case reports, case series, and animal studies. An ideal chelating agent has low toxicity, forms a stable complex with the target metal, has a similar distribution as the metal, and, most importantly, results in a change in clinical outcome. In addition, the chelation agent must prevent the redistribution of metal into the brain.

Central to the discussion of chelation is the understanding of the principles that support this practice. Metals can be described as soft versus hard, and those that are in between these categories are often referred to as borderline. Hard metal ions include sodium and potassium, whereas copper and mercury are often referred to as soft ions because of the large number of electrons around the large ionic radii. Examples of borderline metal ions include lead and zinc. A chelator or ligand such as $CaNa_2EDTA$ contains a carboxyl group that forms the best bond with hard metals, whereas BAL, with its sulfhydryl groups, forms the best bond with soft metal ions.

In the acute setting, chelation therapy often must be instituted based on the clinical scenario alone, because there is often a substantial delay in obtaining the results of a confirmatory metal test. Most available chelators, except $CaNa_2EDTA$, contain thiol groups that are believed to compete with sulfhydryl groups, preventing the inactivation of the numerous sulfhydryl-containing enzymes as well as proteins throughout the body.

Chelators clearly enhance elimination of metals in both animal models and poisoned humans, but whether elimination translates into improved clinical outcomes has not been thoroughly shown. A large multicenter trial tested whether chelation would alter neuropsychological testing in asymptomatic children with moderately increased blood lead concentrations. All children in the study were removed from the source of lead exposure and were randomized to receive either succimer (DMSA) or placebo. Children who received succimer initially had a rapid and significant decrease in their blood lead concentration, but a rebound was observed within 1 week, likely caused by mobilization of lead stores from bone. The placebo group also had a decrease in blood lead concentrations simply from removal of the children from the exposure. At the end of the study period, the 2 groups had statistically similar lead concentrations and there were no proven differences in cognition, behavior, or neuropsychological function. The children treated with succimer had a decrease in growth. Thus, given the lack of benefit, the potential adverse effect on growth and the cost of treatment in this study show that the use of chelation in asymptomatic patients should be viewed with caution. Perhaps the most important intervention performed in the study was the removal of patients from the source of exposure.[79–84]

The use of chelation therapy in chronic metal toxicity is often less clear because diagnosis depends on the clinical presentation as well as proper interpretation of appropriately obtained (nonchallenged) metal testing. **Table 2** contains a list of

Table 2
Chelators currently available in the United States

Dosage/Indication	Adverse Effects

BAL
1. Acute lead encephalopathy
   Dose: 75 mg/m^2 IM every 4 h for 5 days in children and 4 mg/kg every 4 h in adults[a]
2. Acute inorganic arsenic poisoning
   Dose: 3 mg/kg IM every 4 h for 48 h and then twice daily for 7 to 10 d
3. Acute mercury poisoning
   Dose: 5 mg/kg IM initially, followed by 2.5 mg/kg every 12 to 24 h until the patient appears clinically improved (max use is 10 d)
	Lacrimation; emesis; salivation; rhinorrhea; headache; painful injection; injection site sterile abscess; hemolysis in G6PD-deficient patients; chelation of essential metals (prolonged course); dissociation with acidic urine; avoid in patients with peanut allergies

Succimer (DMSA)
1. Mild-moderate lead poisoning (acute or chronic)
   Dose: 350 mg/m^2 in children, 3 times a day for 5 d, followed by 350 mg/m^2 twice a day for 14 d, 10 mg/kg 3 times a day for 5 d, followed by 10 mg/kg twice a day for 14 d in adults
2. Arsenic poisoning
   Dose: 10 mg/kg/dose every 8 h for 5 d
3. Mercury poisoning
   Dose: 10 mg/kg orally 3 times a day for 5 d, then twice a day for 14 d if the gastrointestinal ract is clear
	Gastrointestinal side effects such as diarrhea and emesis; metallic taste; mild increase in liver enzymes; rarely chills, rash, and reversible neutropenia

Prussian Blue
1. Thallium poisoning
   Dose: 9 g divided into 3 g, 3 times per day for adults and 3 g divided into 1 g, 3 times per day for children
2. Cesium poisoning
   Dose: 9 g divided into 3 g, 3 times per day for adults and 3 g divided into 1 g, 3 times per day for children
	Constipation; abdominal pain; discolored (blue) stool

CaNa$_2$EDTA
Sodium EDTA can cause life-threatening hypocalcemia and should not be used
1. Lead encephalopathy
   Dose: 1500 mg/m^2/d approximately 50–75 mg/kg/d by continuous IV infusion, starting 4 h after the first dose of dimercaprol[a]
2. Moderate lead poisoning (BLL of <70 µg/dL)
   Dose: CaNa$_2$EDTA is 1000 mg/m^2/d, approximately 25–50 mg/kg/d in addition to dimercaprol at 50 mg/m^2 every 4 h[b]
	Renal failure; life-threatening hypocalcemia with the use of disodium EDTA; malaise; headache; fatigue; chills or fever; myalgias; anorexia; sneezing; nasal congestion; lacrimation; anemia; transient hypotension; increased prothrombin times

D-Penicillamine (Cuprimine)
1. Lead, mercury, and copper toxicity
   Dose: 1–1.5 g/d given orally in 4 divided doses
   Rarely used because of substantial complications and superior agents
	Allergic reaction (in particular patients allergic to penicillin); aplastic anemia; agranulocytosis; renal failure

Abbreviations: BLL, blood lead level; IM, intramuscular; IV, intravenous.
[a] The first dose of dimercaprol should precede the first dose of CaNa$_2$EDTA by 4 hours to prevent redistribution of lead into the brain.
[b] The use of succimer is typically recommended in these cases.

chelators currently approved in the United States along with indications and adverse effects associated with their use. There are many factors to consider with the use of chelation agents, such as which chelators to choose, and the dose, duration, and frequency. Because most clinicians have negligible experience in treatment, we recommend consultation with a regional poison center and toxicologist.

A subject of current interest involving the use of chelators is the marketing of unapproved chelation drugs by various companies. Despite lack of any evidence for their products, these companies market products as treatments for various disorders such as Parkinson disease, cardiovascular disease, and autism. Targeting patients with long-term chronic disorders, these products are potentially dangerous. An example of this was reported when a child was inappropriately chelated and given edetate disodium rather than $CaNa_2EDTA$. This error caused profound hypocalcemia with resultant death from cardiac arrythmias.[85] These chelation agents come in a variety of forms such as capsules, sprays, and even suppositories. Many companies claim that their products cleanse the body of toxic chemicals and heavy metals. The US Food and Drug Administration (FDA) recently issued a warning to various companies that they may face legal action if they continue to make unsubstantiated claims. Although it is not illegal to sell these products (unless there is clear harm), the FDA can initiate legal actions because of claims to diagnose or treat a disease.

SUMMARY

Metal poisoning represents a complex toxicologic problem that often manifest with a wide range of clinical presentations that may involve multiple organ systems including the nervous system. An awareness of this complex presentation requires knowledge of the varying presentations along with the major forms of metal poisoning: elemental, organic, and inorganic, as well as acute versus chronic time courses. Although chelation therapy remains the cornerstone for the treatment of acute life-threatening poisoning, it should be used to diagnose patients, and its benefit in chronic or low-level toxicity remains unproven.

REFERENCES

1. Duffus JH. "Heavy metals" a meaningless term? (IUPAC Technical Report). Pure Appl Chem 2002;74:793–807.
2. Gaslin MT, Rubin C, Pribitkin EA. Silver nasal sprays: misleading Internet marketing. Ear Nose Throat J 2008;87:217–20.
3. Hori K, Martin TG, Rainey P, et al. Believe it or not silver still poisons! Vet Hum Toxicol 2002;44:291–2.
4. Griffin JP. Famous names: the Esing Bakery, Hong Kong. Adverse Drug React Toxicol Rev 1997;16:79–81.
5. Meggs WJ, Hoffman RS, Shih RD, et al. Thallium poisoning from maliciously contaminated food. J Toxicol Clin Toxicol 1994;32:723–30.
6. Desenclos JC, Wilder MH, Coppenger GW, et al. Thallium poisoning: an outbreak in Florida, 1988. South Med J 1992;85:1203–6.
7. Powell PP. Minamata disease: a story of mercury's malevolence. South Med J 1991;84:1352–8.
8. Ahsan H, Chen Y, Parvez F, et al. Arsenic exposure from drinking water and risk of premalignant skin lesions in Bangladesh: baseline results from the health effects of arsenic longitudinal study. Am J Epidemiol 2006;163:1138–48.
9. Patwardhan JR, Finckh ES. Fatal cadmium-fume pneumonitis. Med J Aust 1976; 1:962–6.

10. Clarkson TW, Magos L, Myers GJ. The toxicology of mercury–current exposures and clinical manifestations. N Engl J Med 2003;349:1731–7.
11. Schultz ST. Does thimerosal or other mercury exposure increase the risk for autism? A review of current literature. Acta Neurobiol Exp (Wars) 2010;70:187–95.
12. Poland GA, Spier R. Fear, misinformation, and innumerates: how the Wakefield paper, the press, and advocacy groups damaged the public health. Vaccine 2010;28:2361–2.
13. Schaffer AW, Pilger A, Engelhardt C, et al. Increased blood cobalt and chromium after total hip replacement. J Toxicol Clin Toxicol 1999;37:839–44.
14. Steens W, von Foerster G, Katzer A. Severe cobalt poisoning with loss of sight after ceramic-metal pairing in a hip-a case report. Acta Orthop 2006;77:830–2.
15. Jacobs JJ, Skipor AK, Patterson LM, et al. Metal release in patients who have had a primary total hip arthroplasty. A prospective controlled, longitudinal study. J Bone Joint Surg Am 1998;80:1447–8.
16. Savory J, Sedor FA. Arsenic poisoning. In: Brown SS, editor. Clinical chemistry and chemical toxicology of metals. New York: Elsevier/North-Holland; 1977. p. 271–86.
17. Krachler M, Zheng J, Emons H. Speciation of antimony for the 21st century: promises and pitfalls. Trends Anal Chem 2001;20:79–90.
18. Lidsky TI, Schneider JS. Lead neurotoxicity in children: basic mechanisms and clinical correlates. Brain 2003;126:5–19.
19. Regan CM. Neural cell adhesion molecules, neuronal development and lead toxicity. Neurotoxicology 1993;14:69–74.
20. Melnick RL, Monti LG, Motzkin SM. Uncoupling of mitochondrial oxidative phosphorylation by thallium. Biochem Biophys Res Commun 1976;69:68–73.
21. Mullins LJ, Moore RD. The movement of thallium ions in muscle. J Gen Physiol 1960;43:759–73.
22. Ibrahim D, Froberg B, Wolf A, et al. Heavy metal poisoning: clinical presentations and pathophysiology. Clin Lab Med 2006;26:67–97.
23. Josephs KA, Ahlskog JE, Klos KJ, et al. Neurologic manifestations in welders with pallidal MRI T1 hyperintensity. Neurology 2005;64:2033–9.
24. Stepens A, Logina I, Liguts V, et al. A parkinsonian syndrome in methcathinone users and the role of manganese. N Engl J Med 2008;358:1009–17.
25. Short AI, Winney RJ, Robson JS. Reversible microcytic hypochromic anaemia in dialysis patients due to aluminum intoxication. Proc Eur Dial Transplant Assoc 1980;17:226–33.
26. Smith EC, Mahurkar SD, Mamdani BH, et al. Diagnosing dialysis dementia. Dial Transplant 1978;7:1264–74.
27. Mendelowitz PC, Hoffman RS, Weber S. Bismuth absorption and myoclonic encephalopathy during bismuth subsalicylate therapy. Ann Intern Med 1990;112:140–1.
28. Monseu G, Struelens M, Roland M. Bismuth encephalopathy. Acta Neurol Belg 1976;76:301–8.
29. Heyman A, Pfeiffer JB, Willett RW. Peripheral neuropathy caused by arsenical intoxication: a study of 41 cases with observations on the effects of BAL (2,3-dimercaptopropanol). N Engl J Med 1956;254:401–9.
30. Chuttani PN, Chawla LS, Sharma TD. Arsenical neuropathy. Neurology 1967;17:269–74.
31. Bank WJ, Pleasure DE, Suzuki K, et al. Thallium poisoning. Arch Neurol 1972;26:456–64.
32. Arbouine MW, Wilson HK. The effect of seafood consumption on the assessment of occupational exposure to arsenic by urinary arsenic speciation measurements. J Trace Elem Electrolytes Health Dis 1992;6:153–60.

33. Brown MJ, Willis T, Omalu B, et al. Deaths resulting from hypocalcemia after administration of edetate disodium: 2003–2005. Pediatrics 2006;118:e534–6.
34. Nagaraj MV, Rao PV, Susarala S. Copper sulphate poisoning, hemolysis and methaemoglobinemia. J Assoc Physicians India 1985;33:308–9.
35. Barbey JT, Pezzullo JC, Soignet SL. Effect of arsenic trioxide on QT interval in patients with advanced malignancies. J Clin Oncol 2003;21:3609–15.
36. Beckman KJ, Bauman JL, Pimental PA, et al. Arsenic-induced torsade de pointes. Crit Care Med 1991;19:290–2.
37. Ortega-Carnicer J, Alcázar R, De la Torre M, et al. Pentavalent antimonial-induced torsade de pointes. J Electrocardiol 1997;30:143–5.
38. Greenberg GN, Levine RJ. Urinary creatinine excretion is not stable: a new method for assessing urinary toxic substance concentrations. J Occup Med 1989 Oct;31:832–8.
39. Sata F, Araki S, Yokoyama K, et al. Adjustment of creatinine-adjusted values in urine to urinary flow rate: a study of eleven heavy metals and organic substances. Int Arch Occup Environ Health 1995;68:64–8.
40. Wagner SL, Weswig P. Arsenic in blood and urine of forest workers as indices of exposure to cacodylic acid. Arch Environ Health 1974;28:77–9.
41. Kersjes MP, Maurer JR, Trestrail JH, et al. An analysis of arsenic exposures referred to the Blodgett Regional Poison Center. Vet Hum Toxicol 1987;29:75–8.
42. Barrett S. Commercial hair analysis. Science or scam? JAMA 1985;254(8):1041–5.
43. Cullen NM, Wolf LR, St Clair D. Pediatric arsenic ingestion. Am J Emerg Med 1995;13:432–5.
44. Barnhart S, Rosenstock L. Cadmium chemical pneumonitis chest 1984;789–91.
45. Czerwinski AW, Ginn HE. Bismuth nephrotoxicity. Am J Med 1964;37:969–75.
46. Reed D, Crawley J, Faro SN, et al. Thallotoxicosis. Acute manifestations and sequelae. JAMA 1963;183:516–22.
47. Goebel HH, Schmidt PF, Bohl J, et al. Polyneuropathy due to acute arsenic intoxication: biopsy studies. J Neuropathol Exp Neurol 1990;49:137–49.
48. Le Quesne PM, McLeod JG. Peripheral neuropathy following a single exposure to arsenic: clinical course in four patients with electrophysiological and histological studies. J Neurol Sci 1977;32:437–51.
49. Cersosimo MG, Koller W. The diagnosis of manganese-induced parkinsonism. Neurotoxicology 2006;27(3):340–6.
50. Arjona A, Mata M, Bonet M. Diagnosis of chronic manganese intoxication by magnetic resonance imaging. N Engl J Med 1997;336:964–5.
51. Needleman HL, Gunnoe C, Leviton A, et al. Deficits in psychological and classroom performance of children with elevated dentine lead levels. N Engl J Med 1979;300:689–95.
52. Young EG, Smith RP. Arsenic content of hair and bone in acute and chronic arsenical poisoning: review of 2 cases examined posthumously from medico-legal aspect. Br Med J 1942;1:251–3.
53. Rosenman KD, Valciukas JA, Glickman L, et al. Sensitive indicators of inorganic mercury toxicity. Arch Environ Health 1986;41:208–15.
54. Whitaker JA, Austin W, Nelson JD. Edathamil calcium disodium (Versenate) diagnostic test for lead poisoning. Pediatrics 1962;29:384–8.
55. Weinberger HL, Post EM, Schneider T, et al. An analysis of 248 initial mobilization tests performed on an ambulatory basis. Am J Dis Child 1987;141:1266–70.
56. Markowitz ME, Rosen JF. Need for the lead mobilization test in children with lead poisoning. J Pediatr 1991;119:305–10.

57. Saenger P, Rosen JF, Markowitz M. Diagnostic significance of edetate disodium calcium testing in children with increased lead absorption. Am J Dis Child 1982; 136:312–5.
58. Markowitz ME, Rosen JF. Assessment of lead stores in children: validation of an 8-hour CaNa$_2$EDTA provocative test. J Pediatr 1984;104:337–41.
59. Sokas RK, Atleson J, Keogh JP. Shortened forms of provocative lead chelation. J Occup Med 1988;30:420–4.
60. Haust HL, Ali H, Haines DS, et al. Short-term administration of dimercaptopropanol (BAL) and calcium disodium edetate (EDTA) for diagnostic and therapeutic lead mobilization. Int J Biochem 1980;12:897–904.
61. Chisolm JJ Jr. Mobilization of lead by calcium disodium edetate. A reappraisal. Am J Dis Child 1987;141:1256–7.
62. Markowitz ME, Bijur PE, Ruff H, et al. Effects of calcium disodium versenate (CaNa$_2$EDTA) chelation in moderate childhood lead poisoning. Pediatrics 1993; 92:265–71.
63. Jugo S, Maliković T, Kostial K. Influence of chelating agents on the gastrointestinal absorption of lead. Toxicol Appl Pharmacol 1975;34:259–63.
64. Chia KS, Tan AL, Chia SE, et al. Renal tubular function of cadmium exposed workers. Ann Acad Med Singapore 1992;21:756–9.
65. Kales SN, Goldman RH. Mercury exposure: current concepts, controversies, and a clinic's experience. J Occup Environ Med 2002;44:143–54.
66. Allain P, Mauras Y, Premel-Cabic A, et al. Effects of an EDTA infusion on the urinary elimination of several elements in healthy subjects. Br J Clin Pharmacol 1991;31:347–9.
67. Allain P, Mauras Y, Krari N, et al. Plasma and urine aluminium concentrations in healthy subjects after administration of sucralfate. Br J Clin Pharmacol 1990;29: 391–5.
68. Allain P, Mauras Y, Chaleil D, et al. Pharmacokinetics and renal elimination of desferrioxamine and ferrioxamine in healthy subjects and patients with haemochromatosis. Br J Clin Pharmacol 1987;24:207–12.
69. Perry HM Jr, Perry EF. Normal concentrations of some trace metals in human urine: changes produced by ethylenediaminetetraacetate. J Clin Invest 1959; 38:1452–63.
70. Frumkin H, Manning CC, Williams PL, et al. Diagnostic chelation challenge with DMSA: a biomarker of long-term mercury exposure? Environ Health Perspect 2001;109:167–71.
71. Soden SE, Lowry JA, Garrison CB, et al. 24-hour provoked urine excretion test for heavy metals in children with autism and typically developing controls, a pilot study. Clin Toxicol (Phila) 2007;45:476–81.
72. Brodkin E, Copes R, Mattman A, et al. Lead and mercury exposures: interpretation and action. CMAJ 2007;176:59–63.
73. Risher JF, Amler SN. Mercury exposure: evaluation and intervention. The inappropriate use of chelating agents in the diagnosis and treatment of putative mercury poisoning. Neurotoxicology 2005;26:691–9.
74. Charlton N, Wallace KL. American College of Medical Toxicology position statement on post-chelator challenge urinary metal testing. J Med Toxicol 2010;6:74–5.
75. Andersen AH. Experimental studies on the pharmacology of activated charcoal. III: adsorption from gastro-intestinal contents. Acta Pharmacol Toxicol 1948;4: 275–84.
76. Lehmann PA, Favari L. Parameters for the adsorption of thallium ions by activated charcoal and Prussian blue. J Toxicol Clin Toxicol 1984;22:331–9.

77. Hoffman RS, Stringer JA, Feinberg RS, et al. Comparative efficacy of thallium adsorption by activated charcoal, Prussian blue, and sodium polystyrene sulfonate. J Toxicol Clin Toxicol 1999;37:833–7.
78. Bailly R, Lauwerys R, Buchet JP, et al. Experimental and human studies on antimony metabolism: their relevance for the biological monitoring of workers exposed to inorganic antimony. Br J Ind Med 1991;48:93–7.
79. Basinger MA, Jones MM. Structural requirements for chelate antidotal efficacy in acute antimony (III) intoxication. Res Commun Chem Pathol Pharmacol 1981;32: 355–63.
80. Zimmer LJ, Carter DE. The efficacy of 2,3-dimercaptopropanol and D-penicillamine on methyl mercury induced neurological signs and weight loss. Life Sci 1978;23:1025–34.
81. Thompson RH, Whittaker VP. Antidotal activity of British anti-Lewisite against compounds of antimony, gold and mercury. Biochem J 1947;41:342–6.
82. Aposhian HV, Carter DE, Hoover TD, et al. DMSA, DMPS, and DMPA–as arsenic antidotes. Fundam Appl Toxicol 1984;4:S58–70.
83. Kreppel H, Reichl FX, Kleine A, et al. Antidotal efficacy of newly synthesized dimercaptosuccinic acid (DMSA) monoesters in experimental arsenic poisoning in mice. Fundam Appl Toxicol 1995;26:239–45.
84. Rogan WJ, Dietrich KN, Ware JH, et al. The effect of chelation therapy with succimer on neuropsychological development in children exposed to lead. N Engl J Med 2001;344:1421–6.
85. Baxter AJ, Krenzelok EP. Pediatric fatality secondary to EDTA chelation. Clin Toxicol (Phila) 2008;46(10):1083–4.

Welding and Parkinsonism

Brent Furbee, MD

KEYWORDS
- Manganism • Manganese • Parkinsonism • Welding • Welders

Welding is the process of joining 2 pieces of metal by applying heat to the edges and melting a welding consumable (welding rod or wire) in the seam between them. In this process, the molten metal from the welding consumable and the edges of the 2 metal pieces forms the weld pool that solidifies to form the joint. The object of this process is to create a weld that is as strong as, or stronger than, the metal pieces being joined. For that reason, manganese is often used in welding consumables in steel welding. It is also present to a lesser degree in the steel itself. Most welding rods and wires used in mild steel welding contain less than 6% manganese. Consumables for high-manganese steel welding and hardfacing may contain considerably higher concentrations. Hardfacing is not welding, but a process used to repair steel surfaces such as blades of earthmoving equipment or high-manganese steel railway equipment. It involves laying down layers of metal on the equipment, which are then ground into the necessary shape. Gouging and cutting of metals also are not considered welding, but involve the heating of metal and result in fumes that are, at times, considerably higher in manganese content than welding fume. Today, multiple industry standards exist to regulate the workplace exposure to welding and manganese fumes.

It has been estimated that more than 5 million workers throughout the world are exposed to welding aerosols each day.[1] For 2008, the Bureau of Labor Statistics reported that 466,400 US workers were employed in jobs engaging them in welding, soldering, and/or brazing.[2] However, among American workers, cases of suspected manganese-induced parkinsonism or manganism are exceedingly rare. Even during the early 1940s with increasing wartime shipbuilding and weapons construction, studies of workers exposed to welding fume failed to show that manganism occurred in the workplace. In a review of the health hazards of electric and gas welders, Britton and Walsh[3] noted that welding rods used outside the United States tended to have higher concentrations of manganese in rod coverings, sometimes approaching 15% to 20%. Regarding US workers, they observed, "Severe manganese poisoning with advanced neurologic findings has not been described."[3]

The author is a paid consultant to the makers of welding consumables.
Indiana Poison Center, Indiana University School of Medicine, B408 Methodist Hospital, Indianapolis, IN 46206, USA
E-mail address: bfurbee@iuhealth.org

MANGANISM AND OCCUPATIONAL EXPOSURES

Long before the concerns regarding a possible association between welding and parkinsonism, there were reports of manganism in manganese grinders, mill workers, and miners. In 1837, John Couper[4] described 2 workers who developed paraplegia in the absence of sensory loss, tremor, or gastrointestinal symptoms. They were removed from work and there was no further progression of symptoms, although they did not improve. Subsequently, 3 more workers developed gait disturbances and were quickly removed from the workplace, after which they recovered.[4]

Toward the latter part of the nineteenth century, more reports of movement and psychiatric disorders among grinders, mill workers, and other handlers of manganese began to surface. Problems included labile affect, speech and writing problems, and particularly, retropulsion and propulsion. Although some of the reported cases were almost certainly misdiagnosed, the similarity was unsettling.[5–7] In 1913, Casamajor[8] reported 9 grinders with comparable findings. He was struck with the similarity to paralysis agitans, which is now known as idiopathic Parkinson disease (IPD).[8]

In 1927, Ashizawa described gross and microscopic findings of an autopsy performed on a 33-year-old brownstone miller who had shown many of the signs and symptoms described in previous reports.[4,7,8] The patient seems to have died of tuberculosis. At autopsy, Ashizawa found that: "The changes in the pallidum were quite remarkable. They consisted of a severe reduction of the gangliocytes of the pars interna, and somewhat less severe in the pars externa..." Intensive changes were also found in the putamen and caudate nucleus, where the degenerative processes were more severe in the large gangliocytes than in the small ones.[9]

In 1954, Parnitzke and Peiffer[10] reviewed autopsy reports of 6 people believed to have had manganism at the time of their deaths. Histopathology from those cases helped to better characterize the central nervous system toxicity of manganese. The investigators identified the basal ganglia, particularly the globus pallidus, as the primary target. The caudate and putamen were also affected.[9–11]

A better recognition of the clinical picture of manganism began to develop as more cases were reported. In 1955, Rodier[12] described 150 manganese miners in Morocco. All of those affected, either drillers or their helpers, worked underground. Workers elsewhere in the mining operation who were also in contact with manganese were not similarly affected. Symptoms most commonly appeared within the first year or two of work. Rodier[12] described a prodromal phase in which the worker would suffer loss of appetite and decreased strength, making even simple tasks difficult. Apathy and a decline in conversation followed. Some workers exhibited an excitatory period that Rodier[12] called manganese psychosis. Some began to behave aggressively. They started to stagger and speech became incoherent. Initial somnolence changed to insomnia. Early increased sexual behavior was followed by impotence.[12]

The intermediate phase was marked by further deterioration of speech and the onset of stuttering. Facial expression took on a dazed expression termed "masque manganique." Some patients seemed euphoric, whereas, less frequently, others experienced spasmodic weeping. The workers moved more slowly and clumsily. Accidents increased and they began having problems eating and drinking.[12]

Muscular hypertonia in extension, particularly in the lower limbs and face, marked the onset of the established phase. Further gait disturbances, as a result of increasing muscle rigidity, led to a roosterlike gate termed pas du coq or cock walk. Those who suffered that affliction would walk on the balls of their feet with ankles extended. Their knees and elbows were held in a flexed position. Walking backward became impossible for many of the affected workers. Tremor was occasionally seen in this stage.

The affected miners in Rodier's[12] study were exposed to manganese concentrations as high as 926 mg/m^3. In contrast, the current Occupational Safety and Health Administration permissible exposure level (PEL) is 5 mg/m^3, which is not to be exceeded at any time. The American Conference of Governmental Industrial Hygienists (ACGIH) threshold limit value (TLV) is 0.2 mg/m^3. This value sets the average exposure that a worker should not exceed during an 8-hour period.

Even in the remarkably poor hygienic conditions of the time, these cases represented only a small portion of the workers in a given operation. In 1965, Abd El Naby and Hassanein[13] reported 45 miners in Egypt with clinical features of manganism. The investigators noted: "Even if we make allowance for those patients who have been missed or wrongly diagnosed, it would appear that this type of poisoning is still a rarity in this country."

In December of 1984, the owner of a ferromanganese smelter in Taiwan removed the malfunctioning ventilation system in his factory to replace it.[14] Smelting operations continued while the installation of the new system was delayed. In October of 1985, a 44-year-old worker from that facility presented with clumsiness, rigidity, bradykinesia, masklike face, and micrographia. Parkinsonism was diagnosed and manganese was suspected as the cause. Clinical investigation of his coworkers revealed 5 other patients with similar symptoms. All of the patients had worked in an area above the furnace where manganese concentrations usually exceeded 28.8 mg/m^3 and increased to even higher concentrations for 30 minutes a day.[14] The patients had been discovered in a 20-month period when the ventilation system was not working properly or was absent. Four of the patients' coworkers from that area were asymptomatic. In the rest of the factory, where concentrations were generally less than 1.5 mg/m^3, no cases were found among the remaining 126 workers.[15] When the ventilation system was repaired, the highest manganese concentration was 4.4 mg/m^3. No cases were subsequently reported. Of the 6 original patients, 1 died and 1 was lost to follow-up. Magnetic resonance imaging (MRI) was normal in 3 of the remaining 4 patients with manganism; however, those studies were performed several years after their presentation.[16] The patients also received 6-fluorodopa positron emission tomography (PET) scans that showed normal striatal uptake, making IPD an unlikely diagnosis.

In 1993, Huang and colleagues[17] stated: "The order of occurrence of neurologic symptoms in these six patients was determined. The most frequent initial symptom was gait disturbance especially walking backward. Patients tended to fall because of freezing in turning. Writing difficulty and hypophonia were the next initial symptoms in chronologic order of onset. Fatigue and muscle cramps were also frequent." Muscle stiffness, fatigue, sleep disturbance, walking backward, freezing during turning, and writing tended to worsen, whereas tremor showed improvement. In contrast, patients with IPD commonly have a pill-rolling resting tremor with a frequency of 3 to 7 Hz that sometimes worsens with progression of their disease. Tremor is not a prominent feature of manganism and, when it occurs, it is usually a more subtle postural tremor with high frequency and low amplitude. As seen in Wilson disease, dystonic gait (cock's gait), foot and facial dystonia may occur with manganism. None of the 4 patients with manganism improved with L-dopa therapy.[18]

In 1998, Huang and colleagues[16] reported a 10-year follow-up of the 4 surviving patients. The most prominent progression of symptoms was found in gait disturbance, rigidity, foot tapping speed, and writing. In 2003, Huang[19] reported: "The neurologic manifestations included micrographia, masked facies, hypophonia or stuttering speech, dystonia; gait en bloc, difficulty in walking especially backward, postural instability, and rigidity. All of the patients did not have resting tremor except for patient 4 who had tongue tremor while stretching out his tongue."

The patients underwent a [99m]-Tc-TRODAT-1 (single-photon emission computed tomography) scan that showed significantly higher uptake of a cocaine analogue than did patients with IPD. [99m]-Tc-TRODAT-1 can bind specifically to the dopamine transporter (DAT) sites on presynaptic dopamine neuron terminals. The investigators suggested that might be a better tool for differentiating manganism from IPD.[19]

These reports of clinical and radiologic findings added significantly to the growing body of information about the presentation and progression of manganism. Both IPD and manganism may show bradykinesia, rigidity, and postural instability, but there are several factors that help differentiate manganism from IPD or other forms of parkinsonism.

Manganism	IPD
Clinical Presentation	
Symmetric onset and symptoms	Asymmetrical onset and symptoms
Retropulsion, propulsion	Less pronounced
Cock walk	Infrequent
No resting tremor, occasional postural tremor	Resting pill-rolling tremor
Hypophonia	Less common
Micrographia	Less common
MRI	
Bilateral T1-weighted hyperintensities in globus pallidus	Normal
Fluorodopa PET	
Normal	Decreased striatal uptake especially in the posterior putamen
Pathology	
Neurodegeneration of the globus pallidus	Neurodegeneration of substantia nigra
Lewy bodies absent	Lewy bodies present
Response to levodopa	
Transient improvement, motor complications uncommon	Sustained improvement, motor complications common

The diagnosis of manganism requires a preponderance of findings. For example, symmetry of symptoms favors manganism, but asymmetry may occur, particularly with dystonia.[13,16] The presence or absence of a single finding cannot be used to absolutely establish or rule out the diagnosis.

Case Reports in Welders

In 1932, Erich Beintker,[20] a Senior Industrial Medical Officer, reported 2 welders with various health problems thus raising the question of an association with electric arc welding.

One worker had been welding for about 4 years inside boilers and tanks. Except for eye protection, no other protective measures were taken. He complained of dizziness, loss of appetite, occasional vomiting, productive cough, night sweats, erectile dysfunction, and insomnia. He was noted to have a fine tremor but there was no detailed examination of the nervous system.

A second worker had welded for 10 years in boilers and containers. During that time he was involved in an accidental spill of molten iron into his right ear. His speech was hesitant and he stuttered. He was noted to have a marked Romberg sign, but no ataxia or significant impairment walking with closed eyes.

Beintker[20] measured the content of manganese in the welding electrodes and concluded that the workers symptoms were caused by a mild form of manganese poisoning. Neither welder had symptoms that indicated parkinsonism; some of their symptoms appeared more likely to have been caused by other illness such as heart disease and a middle ear injury. Serum, blood, or urine manganese concentrations were not obtained nor were air concentrations available to document exposure.[20]

In a review of literature to 2005, McMillan[21] noted that there had been 24 published reports listing 45 persons classified as welders who had been diagnosed with clinical manganism. The author stated that, on review, this probably represented a total of 29 true welders. That designation excluded nonwelding activities such as cutting, gouging, and hardfacing. The following cases have been selected from those because they are the most commonly cited in related literature.

Oltramare and colleagues[22] reported 2 welders working in a large French Swiss structural steel firm who presented after more than 25 years of welding. They both worked in enclosed areas with limited ventilation. Their only protection was the welding shield that they wore. Manganese air concentrations were as high as 125 mg/m^3 at times.[22] Their complaints included vertigo, profuse sweating, fine tremor, dysequilibrium, retropulsion, hyperreflexia, and loss of libido. The investigators noted that the presentation of both workers was "mainly subjective" and "not very characteristic." They then tested the neuromuscular excitability of the 2 welders and compared it with 10 of their cohorts. Based on these tests, they diagnosed chronic manganese poisoning.[22]

Nelson and colleagues[23] reported a 44-year-old arc welder of 25 years. He had been responsible for the repair and recycling of railroad track, which was made of steel containing 11% to 14% Mn. For 15 years before the onset of symptoms, he had worked indoors without an exhaust system. He engaged in cutting of 20% Mn alloy, and it seems likely that his work included hardfacing. He became more irritable and tearful. His memory was impaired and cognitive function declined. He had frequent falls and difficulty walking downhill. His symptoms were more pronounced on the right at the time of onset and he was noted to have a right hemisensory deficit. MRI showed hyperintensity of the globi pallidi on T-1 weighted images.[23]

Discalzi and colleagues[24] reported a 53-year-old Italian worker who noted a postural tremor, bradykinesia, and hypertonia in the summer of 1996. A year later, an MRI showed bilateral symmetric hyperintensity of the globus pallidus and substantia nigra on T1-weighted images. The patient was seen by the investigators 2 years after onset of symptoms. They considered that, by virtue of working in electrode fixation, he was likely exposed to higher manganese concentrations. He also worked in confined spaces during his employment as a ship welder. Removal from exposure and chelation with CaNa$_2$ edetate (calcium disodium EDTA) were associated with a decrease in symptoms. On follow-up in June of 1999, "tremor had almost disappeared and gait appeared normal." Fluorodopa PET scan was not reported.[24]

Sato and colleagues[25] reported a 56-year-old Japanese ship welder with 30-years' experience who developed postural instability and dysgraphia. He had bradykinesia, rigidity, masklike expression, dystonia, and postural reflex impairment. His MRI showed hyperintensity of the globi pallidi, dentate nucleus, midbrain, tegmentum, pontis, and cerebral white matter on T1-weighted images. The investigators stated that the diagnosis of manganese poisoning was "based upon increased manganese concentrations in blood and urine and on the marked increase of urinary manganese levels after administration of a chelating agent." Although the urine manganese concentration rose after chelation, the patient did not improve. Administration of L-dopa/carbidopa led to an improvement in his bradykinesia, muscular rigidity, dysbasia, and retropulsion. Improvement following dopamine agonists is suggestive of IPD as opposed to manganism.[25]

Ono and colleagues[26] reported a 17-year-old Japanese boy who had welded for 2 years when he presented with complaints of involuntary movement of the right upper and lower extremities. He was noted to have decreased muscle tone in the affected side. Involuntary movement was most pronounced in the right shoulder, arm, and the right lower portion of his face. Finger to nose and diadochokinesis were also impaired on the right. Blood manganese was increased at 4.3 μg/dL (0.8–2.5 μg/dL). Bilateral hyperintensity of the globus pallidus extended to the cerebral peduncle on T1-weighted images of his MRI. Myoclonic activity decreased after admission and further decreased after 5 days of treatment with Ca-EDTA. Two days following chelation, his MRI had improved and his blood manganese concentration subsequently fell within the reference range. The investigators note that he "showed myoclonic involuntary movement (IVM), but no parkinsonism."[26]

Sadek and colleagues[27] reported a 33-year-old American welder who presented with a 2-year progression of cognitive slowing, rigidity, and postural/movement tremor of the right hand. During his 2 years of welding, he had often worked in the false hold of ships where he welded without respiratory equipment. He had taken Sinemet for 2 months without improvement. His family history was positive for a maternal great aunt with Parkinson disease. His Mini-Mental State Examination (MMSE) was normal. Neurologic examination revealed slowed saccadic eye movement and hypomimia. He had mild cogwheel rigidity of the upper extremities that was more pronounced on the right. A low-amplitude action tremor was evident in the right arm. His gait was mildly broad-based, fast paced, and stiff. He was also noted to walk on his toes, which the investigators characterized as a cock-walk gait. Laboratory studies included a serum manganese concentration of 22.9 μg/L (8.0–18.7μg/L) obtained 4 weeks after cessation of welding. MRI showed hyperintensity of the basil ganglia on T1-weighted images. Levodopa/carbidopa therapy produced no noticeable improvement. Bowler and colleagues[28] reported a follow-up of this patient.

Kenangil and colleagues[29] reported a 32-year-old Turkish man who had welded for 10 years when, at the age of 29 years, he developed mild postural instability and bradykinesia that progressed. Neurologic examination showed "mild hypomimia, bilateral symmetric bradykinesia and rigidity, mild dystonia in the right foot, and postural instability. He had dystonic gait (cock's walk) strutting on the toes prominently on the right foot with plantar flexion and inversion accompanied by extension and abduction posture of the arms." His MRI showed symmetric increased signal intensity of the globus pallidus bilaterally on T1-weighted images. He did not respond to levodopa or pramipexole therapy. Occupational history indicated that, during welding, he had not worn a mask or respiratory equipment and worked in closed and crowded space. He denied drug exposure that could have caused extrapyramidal effects.[29]

PATHOPHYSIOLOGY

The mechanism by which manganese causes parkinsonism continues to be studied. The primary target organs are the globus pallidus internus, striatum, and substantia nigra pars reticulata. The caudate and putamen may be affected to a lesser degree, whereas the substantia nigra pars compacta, the primary target of IPD, is spared.

Several theories exist regarding the exact cellular injury but most involve the production of reactive oxygen species and damage to mitochondria in glial cells. Thus, manganism does not seem to be a result of decreased dopamine production as seen in IPD. That is consistent with the observation that therapy intended to increase dopamine production is not beneficial in patients with manganism.

PHARMACOKINETICS OF MANGANESE

Only 3% to 5% of ingested manganese is absorbed. Manganese-rich foods include grains, nuts, tea, and legumes. The daily dietary intake ranges from 2 to 5 mg, with some macrobiotic diets exceeding 10 mg/d.[30] An essential element for humans, manganese is necessary for several enzymes including arginase, glutamine synthetase, and superoxide dismutase, which is an important antioxidant mitochondrial enzyme. Although no clear syndrome exists for manganese deficiency in humans, manganese excess in sufficient quantities can lead to manganese-induced parkinsonism (manganism).

Occupational exposures are primarily via inhalation. Historically, mining, grinding, and smelting have been most frequently associated with manganism; however, concern has risen in recent years about the possible risk to other occupations where manganese exposure occurs including welding. Speciation, solubility, and particle size influence inhalation absorption. Metals can occur in different chemical physical or morphologic states representing various species of that metal. Speciation also influences solubility as is seen with manganese chloride ($MnCl_2$) compared with the less soluble (and therefore less absorbable) manganese dioxide (MnO_2). Roels and colleagues[31] showed significantly less gastrointestinal absorption of MnO_2 compared with $MnCl_2$. The particle size of dust or fume is also an important factor in inhalation absorption. Some particles are too large to be inhaled, or are trapped in mucous lining the trachea. Most particles greater than 1 μm tend to localize at or near the carina. Approximately 20% of respirable particles are deposited in the alveoli, and a significant number are consumed by macrophages which are then removed via the mucociliary escalator, coughed from the pulmonary tree, and swallowed.

In contrast with manganese oxide, which is produced in mining and grinding of manganese, the combustion of welding consumables produces fume particles that can be irregular or spherical in shape. They commonly occur as aggregates of metals that exist as long chains up to several micrometers in length, or lacelike structures, both of which may occur in clusters. Although miners and grinders most frequently encounter manganese oxide, which is more readily absorbed, welders are exposed to oxygen-containing particles (spinels) that include combinations of metals such as Fe-Mn oxide.[32]

Elements that may be found in welding fume include iron, sodium, chromium, molybdenum, potassium, oxygen, and manganese. Iron compounds constitute the largest proportion of mild steel welding fume. Silicon is also an important component in spherical particles. These particles have a core consisting of a conglomeration of metals surrounded by a silicon shell. Iron accounts for the highest metal concentration in these particles.[33–35]

About 80% of absorbed manganese is bound to globulin and albumin. It is distributed primarily to the liver and kidney.[36] A small portion is bound, in its trivalent form, to transferrin. Several mechanisms have been proposed regarding the entry of manganese into the brain, including diffusion,[37] divalent metal transporter 1 (DMT-1), ZIP8, and transferrin.[38] Some animal studies have suggested that the mechanism of manganese entry into the brain may be saturable.[39,40] It seems that diffusion is the most common route of transfer out of the brain.[41]

Manganese is eliminated in a biphasic fashion. Following exposure, the early elimination is rapid, with a $T_{1/2}$ of about 4 days before it markedly slows to a $T_{1/2}$ of about 39 days.[42] The early phase eliminates nearly 35% of an administered dose, whereas the late phase accounts for approximately 65%. If predose exposure has been ongoing, the $T_{1/2}$ of the early phase is decreased to 1.5 days, indicating that ongoing exposure increases elimination rates.[43] Early studies of excretion showed that ongoing manganese exposure increases the rate of clearance.[44] Dastur and colleagues[45] showed that injected radiolabeled Mn remained in the brain in animals sacrificed at 278 days. Newland and colleagues[46] showed that half-lives in the primate head (perhaps reflecting bone retention) ranged from 223 to 267 days following exposure.

Mn enters serum as Mn^{2+} where some of it is reversibly bound to α_2-macroglobulin. Both free divalent manganese and the Mn-α_2-macroglobulin complex are rapidly cleared by the liver (minutes to hours). There, a small portion is oxidized to Mn^{3+}. In its trivalent state, that manganese can complex with transferrin. The transferrin complex is cleared more slowly.[47] Borg and Cotzias[48] found that plasma Mn concentrations decreased to statistically insignificant levels in 1 to 2 days following injection of $^{54}MnCl_2$ in humans. Total blood concentrations reached their nadir at that point, but then increased for longer than 50 days thereafter. Blood taken from a patient 66 days after injection of $^{54}MnCl_2$ contained almost the entire radioactivity in the red cell fraction. The amount in the initial plasma samples was considerably more than 10 times that in packed red cells but, in 1 to 2 days, when it had dropped precipitously, the red blood cell (RBC) radioactivity began to increase. This finding seems to reflect the rapid clearance of Mn or its redistribution into tissues. The increase in RBC manganese continued for several days as it was incorporated into newly forming RBCs.[48] Thus, plasma concentrations are of little use because they decrease so rapidly following exposure. RBC concentrations, and those of whole blood, are a better reflection of ongoing exposure. In the absence of further exposure, those concentrations begin to decrease with RBC destruction as older cells hemolyse with time.

NEUROPSYCHOLOGICAL STUDIES

Although clinical features of manganism are straightforward, researchers have, for several years, attempted to identify prodromal indicators that herald its onset. Concern has been raised that low doses of inhaled manganese might, in time, cause the same clinical picture that was seen in past cases of much greater exposure. In 1837, Couper[4] recognized that manganese grinders who had difficulty walking were at risk of developing the progression of symptoms that came to be known as manganism. Subsequently, less obvious features of manganism such as micrographia and hypophonia were identified. The advent of neuropsychological testing has given rise to several studies in the last 3 decades in workers exposed to manganese. In the mid 1980s, Roels and colleagues[49] studied 141 workers in an Mn plant in Belgium producing salt and oxide. They were compared with 104 nonexposed workers and it was found that, on neurologic examination, there was no difference. Neuropsychological testing showed that the workers performed worse than controls on eye-hand coordination, hand steadiness, short-term memory, and simple reaction time. In a study published in 1999, they revisited those workers and reported that since removal from the environment, their eye-hand coordination had significantly improved, but hand steadiness and visual reaction time had not improved after at least 3 years without Mn exposure.[50] Crump and Rousseau[51] also studied that population and concluded that there was no indication that the changes observed by Roels and colleagues[49,50] had progressed in the subsequent 11 years.

One of the frequently cited studies by proponents of welding-induced parkinsonism is that of Racette and colleagues.[52] The investigators identified 15 welders with parkinsonism from their movement disorder clinic in St Louis from 953 new parkinsonian patients seen between 1996 and 2000; 2 control groups were selected. One hundred patients who were diagnosed with IPD were sequentially ascertained from their Movement Disorders Clinic. The second group consisted of 6 patients with IPD, from the same center, who were age and gender matched to the welders. Fluorodopa PET studies were performed on 2 of the welders and 13 subjects with typical IPD. The investigators stated: "Welders were younger at symptom onset (46 years; range 29 to 68) compared with sequentially ascertained controls 63 years: range, 30 to 81; $P<.0001$ who had a typical age at onset."[52]

Of the welders, 53% had a family history of IPD, compared with 41% and 32% in the control groups. Thirteen of the 15 welders had significant improvement with levodopa treatment. The investigators assert that "parkinsonism associated with welding is not clinically different from IPD with the exception of a younger age at onset." It could be argued that these were patients with IPD who coincidently were welders. The investigators concluded that welding fume (but not necessarily manganese) produced a clinical picture that only differed from IPD in that it had an earlier age of onset, and might serve as an accelerant for IPD.[52]

Racette and colleagues[53] studied a group of 1950 welding claimants from August 2002 and March 2003. They reported on 1423 welders from that group who resided in Alabama. A pseudorandom selection of 112 subjects was tested for rigidity and Unified Parkinson Disease Rating Scale motor subsection 3 (UPDRS3) was performed. They then were given a questionnaire concerning medical and employment history. They were videotaped during the UPDRS3. They were then rated by movement disorder fellows who were aware that most were litigants. Definite Parkinson disease (PD) or probable PD subjects were determined from the 1423 welders and the prevalence of PD was compared with that of Copiah Co, Mississippi, where a previous study of the prevalence of parkinsonism was performed in 1985. Of that group, using liberal criteria, they found that 148 subjects had definite PD (10.4%) and 185 had probable PD (13.0%). With regard to prevalence comparisons and the relationship between exposure and parkinsonism, the investigators state: "In univariate logistic regression analysis, higher exposure was associated with the diagnosis of parkinsonism using the conservative (OR = 1.025, 95% CI 0.942 to 1.116) and liberal (OR = 1.015, 95% CI 0.934 to 1.103) criteria."[53] Neither of those odds ratios (ORs) achieves statistical significance and, even if they did, they would be so low that they would not be convincing of an effect given that type of study. They further state: "However, when age was included in the regression equation, only age remained associated with definite PD ($P<.0001$) using both sets of criteria. Age was modestly correlated with exposure ($r = 0.297$, $P<.001$). There was no significant correlation between UPDRS3 score and welding hours for the entire sample or in the active welders."[53]

Bowler and colleagues[54] studied 47 welders, noting mental, medical, and neurologic complaints that prompted their referral for evaluation. Ambient air measurements of the welding sites, personal exposure monitoring, MRI, and biomarkers of exposure to manganese were not available.

Forty-six controls were taken from a 2001 study in munitions workers by one of the investigators. They had been chosen at random in another state. The welders had been referred by 2 neurologists who were examining these and other welders for participation in a legal action. Tests were administered for cognition, information processing, memory, visuomotor and visuospatial skills, verbal skills, and motor skills. The investigators report statistically significant ORs for information processing, some working memory, visuomotor tracking speed, and motor skills. They did not show statistical significance for some working memory or any cognitive flexibility or verbal skills. Welders had statistically significant increases in reporting of symptoms including headache and chemical sensitivity, visual and sensory problems, dermatologic, and gastrointestinal problems, and neurologic, memory, anxiety, depression, and sleep disorders.[54]

In 2007, Bowler and colleagues[55] revisited 43 Bay Bridge workers who were previously studied and used a large battery of neuropsychological tests and self-reported symptoms that were then compared with their whole blood and cumulative exposure index. Except for olfactory tests, no control group was used. Cognitive deficits were found in 79% of the welders.[55] From the 43 Bay Bridge workers, Bowler and colleagues[55,56] identified 11 workers as having manganism based on complaints or findings including:

Sleep disturbance
Slurred speech
Bradykinesia
Monotonous voice
Mood changes
Muscular rigidity
Hallucinations
Tremors
Headaches
Facial masking
Postural instability
Olfaction loss
Sexual dysfunction.

The diagnosis was made from 3 criteria:

1. Bay Bridge welding or 6 or more months with 3 or more years previous welding
2. Three or more self-reported symptoms associated with Mn exposure
3. At least 1 of the asymmetric features or a score of >2 on 2 different Unified PD Rating Scale (UPDRS) motor areas.

For the UPDRS used, a normal subject can score up to 3. The 11 welders scored lower on the neuropsychological testing than norms of the general population. There was no control group. They were then compared with whole blood Mn concentrations and cumulative exposure index (CEI). When adjusted for blood Mn, welders performed worse on cognitive flexibility and visuospatial domains. When adjusted for dose, they performed worse on attention/concentration/working memory domain and verbal learning/auditory perception domain.[56]

Zoni and colleagues[57] reviewed 31 studies including 18 occupational, 7 environmental, and 6 involving children. Some welding studies were included. The most reported tests from these studies were simple reaction time, finger tapping, digit symbol, and digit span. The investigators concluded that motor function and mood were most affected in adults. They also noted: "Although the disparity of the tests administered makes the comparison quite difficult, some useful indication can be drawn from the existing literature. Not all the studies showed coherent results, even while using the same and most sensitive tests."[57]

Meyer-Baron and colleagues[58] performed a meta-analysis of 13 studies measuring cognitive and motor performance in 958 exposed workers, some of whom were welders, but most were from other occupations. Two-thirds of the findings in the studies failed to reach statistical significance. The investigators concluded: "The analysis provided consistent evidence of lower cognitive and motor performance associated with exposure to Mn." They found inhaled manganese more predictive of decreased function.[58]

Greiffenstein and Lees-Haley[59] performed a meta-analysis of 41 variables in 19 studies and found that: "Tasks with the highest effect size (ES) included clerical substitution tasks, digit span, tapping endurance, and Swedish Performance Evaluation System "Additions" reaction time, but none exceeded the ES for education or aptitude." They further concluded that the data did not support a theory of preclinical (early) neuromotor or cognitive dysfunction.[59]

Advances in neurobehavioral testing have produced more numerous and complex tests but have also led to more diverse and confusing results. Greiffenstein and Lees-Haley[59] observed: "The Mn-cognition literature to date shows substantially conflicting results. Studies differ widely in neuropsychological tasks selected, the total number of measures, sample size, subject demographics, cultural context, subjective versus objective data, amount of exposure, industrial context, and weak/normal neuropsychological patterns."[59]

EPIDEMIOLOGIC STUDIES

Several epidemiologic studies have attempted to address the risk of IPD, other forms of parkinsonism, and various neurologic diseases in a wide range of occupations and environmental settings. The following are some of the commonly referenced studies.

Fryzek and colleagues[60] retrospectively evaluated rates of hospitalizations for neurodegenerative disorders in Danish metal manufacturing workers. They studied 27,839 male Danish workers engaged in manufacturing of metal goods in Denmark. The National Supplementary Pension Fund data on workers were used for additional data. It links with hospitals for admissions. The companies were visited in 1986 to determine those workers who were exposed to welding. Shipbuilding workers were excluded. Questionnaires were mailed to the 90% of that group who were still alive in 1986. Questions included smoking history and working conditions. Of the 9817, 8190 (83%) responded. ICD8 and ICD10 codes were used to note PD, degenerative diseases of basal ganglia, dystonia, other extrapyramidal and movement disorders, and other forms of parkinsonism.[60]

For each neurologic disorder, a standardized disease-specific hospitalization rate ratio (SHR; ie, observed/expected cases of disease) was calculated. Subjects were compared with the general population of Denmark with regard to hospitalization rates. The investigators concluded: "…this cohort of Danish welders with more than 20 years of systematic follow-up had rates of PD and other neurologic conditions consistent with those of the general population of Denmark."[60]

Park and colleagues[61] reviewed death certificate information for all deaths in 22 states between the years of 1992 and 1998. Data were obtained from the National Occupational Mortality Surveillance System, which includes occupation or business/industry. Cause of death was coded to ICD9 codes. A case was defined by any mention on the death certificate of presenile dementia, Alzheimer disease, and PD or motor neuron disease. Controls were those without neurologic disease. For welding they found: "Of the four neurodegenerative diseases under study, only PD was associated with occupations where arc welding of steel is performed and only for the 20 PD deaths below age 65 MOR = 1.77, 95% CI = 1.08–2.75."

However, for welders of all ages, the mortality ORs (MORs) for motor neuron disease and PD were 0.66 and 0.87 and were statistically significant. The rates of presenile dementia and Alzheimer disease were decreased, but not statistically significant.[61]

Fored and colleagues[62] studied the association between employment as a welder and all basal ganglia and movement disorders. They identified 49,488 men recorded as welders or flame cutters in the 1960 or 1970 Swedish National Census. They then compared that cohort's rate of specific basal ganglia and movement disorders between 1964 and 2003 with 489,572 gainfully employed men from the general population who were age and geographically matched. They used a survey from 1974 to 1975 of workplace air pollutant concentrations to estimate exposure. They identified 403 welders and flame cutters with basal ganglia or movement disorders, of whom 353 were diagnosed with PD, 44 with secondary parkinsonism, 21 with other degenerative disease of the basal ganglia, 4 with dystonia, and 26 with other extrapyramidal and movement disorders. No cases of poisoning caused by manganese and its compounds were observed. The investigators concluded:

"This well defined, large, nationwide cohort study of Swedish welders with up to 40 years of follow-up did not reveal any statistically significantly increased risks for Parkinson's disease or other basal ganglia and movement disorders for welders compared with an age and geographically matched general population comparison cohort."[62]

Other epidemiologic studies have failed to show an increased risk of manganism, IPD, or other basal ganglia diseases in welders.[63–65] The studies cited earlier were chosen as representative of the controversy concerning welding and the development of parkinsonism. Neurobehavioral studies have been criticized for study design and the inclusion of claimants or litigants as subjects.[54,56,66] Some epidemiologic studies have also been faulted for design[67] and for some being funded by industries involved in welding.[60,62,64,65]

TESTING

Although the primary means of clearance of manganese is via the gut, some is excreted in urine. The urinary concentration of manganese in the general population varies among different laboratories but ranges from 1 to 10 μg/L.[68] Specimens collected following chelation can show a dramatic increase in manganese concentration even in the absence of increased exposure.[69–71] Urine manganese is considered a poor marker for manganese exposure and is not an indication of toxicity.

Because about 85% of manganese is incorporated in RBCs, serum manganese concentrations are not reliable markers of exposure beyond a few days. Reference ranges vary among different laboratories but serum concentrations in the general population usually range from 0.9 to 2.9 μg/L.[72] The clearance of manganese from serum is rapid, whereas clearance from whole blood, because of Mn stored in RBCs, is much slower since its elimination requires destruction of the RBC. Therefore, whole blood or RBC manganese concentrations are considered a better reflection of manganese exposures in a longer time period.[42] Whole blood concentrations of manganese, measured by 3 current reference laboratories, range from 4.2 to 18.7 μg/L.[73–75]

MRI can show manganese deposition in the brain and other organs. In the brain, it appears as bilateral hyperintensity of the globus pallidus on T1-weighted images. Hyperintensity has also been reported in the caudate, putamen, and substantia nigra (SN). Although MRI may not distinguish which part of the SN is affected, pathologic changes seem to be limited to the pars reticulata.[76] However, hyperintensity of the globi pallidi can be seen with disorders that do not involve manganese depositions. Those disorders include Fahr disease (hypoparathyroidism/pseudohypoparathyroidism), nonketotic hyperglycemic episodes, hamartomas of neurofibromatosis type 1, hypoxic-ischemic encephalopathy of hemorrhage caused by Japanese encephalitis,[77] iron deposition in Hallervorden-Spatz disease, and copper deposition in Wilson disease. Fat deposition, hemoglobin breakdown products, melanoma and calcification, methemoglobin associated with intracerebral bleeding, or hemorrhagic infarction can also cause hyperintensities on MRI, although they are usually unilateral.[23,77]

Manganese deposition in the globus pallidus can occur in patients with liver failure because of their inability to eliminate it via the biliary route.[78,79] On rare occasions, patients receiving chronic parenteral hyperalimentation, which contains manganese as a supplement, have also shown this finding.[80,81] More recently, illicit use of ephedrone (methcathinone), which uses potassium permanganate in its manufacturing, has been reported to cause MRI findings and manganism.[82,83] However, this finding reflects exposure but is not diagnostic of toxicity. Dietz and colleagues[84] found that MRI findings correlated with MnO_2 exposure in 90 workers but did not predict neurologic impairment. Kim and colleagues[85] studied welders, smelters, and welding rod manufacturing workers. Among the 38 welders, 73.5% had hyperintensities of the globus pallidus on MRI, but none had symptoms of manganism. This finding led the investigators to conclude that concentrations of manganese required to cause MRI changes are lower than those needed to cause manganism. Hyperintensity may resolve within a few months to 2 years or longer[29,86,87] and, therefore, its absence does not necessarily rule out manganism in someone with a consistent clinical picture.[88,89]

Some investigators have studied the pallidal index as an indicator of manganese exposure and poorer performance on neurobehavioral tests.[90,91] That index represents the ratio of the globus pallidus to subcortical frontal white matter signal intensity on T1-weighted sagittal images of the brain.

TREATMENT

Manganism is poorly responsive to therapy. Patients who are removed from exposure early may have a better chance of improvement.[4] Chelation with EDTA has been used with mixed results in patients suspected to have manganism.[92] It has yet to be established as beneficial in manganese toxicity. The administration of chelating agents does increase metal excretion in patients. Because manganese exposure is ubiquitous, it is not surprising that increased urinary excretion of manganese and other metals follows administration of agents such as EDTA. Urinary excretion of Mn following Ca-EDTA administration to patients without any exposure history has been shown to increase urinary manganese many times over within a few hours of administration.[69-71] Appropriate collection of specimens is essential in accurate determination of Mn concentrations because contamination can significantly increase concentrations.

SUMMARY

Manganism is a clinical diagnosis based on a preponderance of findings that establish the presence of parkinsonism, but separate it from IPD and other forms. Laboratory findings are of marginal help. MRI may help confirm exposure, but does not establish disease. Ancillary studies such as fluorodopa PET may help rule out other diseases such as IPD. Exposure alone is also insufficient to confirm the diagnosis. Of cases presented in the medical literature, those most consistent with the diagnosis seem to have been exposed to high concentrations of manganese in poorly ventilated areas with little or no protective gear.

Manganism is parkinsonism. It is not a subclinical disease. Efforts to identify subclinical signs that would predict the onset of manganism will be, and should be, continued but, to date, neurobehavioral studies have not identified a clear seminal indicator of manganism. Epidemiologic studies have failed to show that welders are at increased risk for parkinsonism, but that does not rule out the possibility that an individual can develop manganism following intense exposure. However, those studies do indicate that such an occurrence would be rare.

REFERENCES

1. Antonini JM, Stone S, Roberts JR, et al. Effect of short-term stainless steel welding fume inhalation exposure on lung inflammation, injury, and defense responses in rats. Toxicol Appl Pharmacol 2007;223(3):234–45.
2. Bureau of Labor Statistics, Welding, soldering, and brazing workers, in Occupational Outlook Handbook. 2010–2011, U.S. Department of Labor. Available at: http://www.bls.gov/oco/ocos226.htm. Accessed April 28, 2011.
3. Britton J, Walsh E. Health hazards of electric and gas welding. J Ind Hyg Toxicol 1940;22:125–51.
4. Couper J. On the effects of black oxide of manganese when inhaled into the lungs. British Annals of Medicine and Pharmacology, Vital Statistics and General Science 1837;I:41–2.
5. Edsall D, Wilbur P, Drinker C. The occurrence, course, and prevention of chronic manganese poisoning. J Indust Hyg 1919;1:183.
6. Embden H. Zur Kenntnis der metalischen Nervengifte (Ueber die chronische Manganveriftung der Braunsteinmuller). Deutsch Med Wehnschr 1901;27:795 [in French].
7. Von Jaksch R. On manganese toxicoses and manganese phobia. Munch Med Wochenschr 1907;20:969–72.
8. Casamajor L. An unusual form of mineral poisoning affecting the nervous system: manganese? JAMA 1913;60(9):646–9.
9. Ashizawa R. Autopsy report on a case involving chronic manganese poisoning. Japanese J Med Sci VII 1930;I:173–91.
10. Parnitzke K, Peiffer J. On the characteristics and pathological anatomy of chronic manganese poisoning. Arch Psych Neurol Disord (J Neurol Psychiatry) 1954;192: 404–29.
11. Canavan M, Cobb S, Drinker C. Chronic manganese poisoning. Arch Neurol 1934;32:501–13.
12. Rodier J. Manganese poisoning in Moroccan miners. Br J Ind Med 1955;12(1):21–35.
13. Abd el Naby S, Hassanein M. Neuropsychiatric manifestations of chronic manganese poisoning. J Neurol Neurosurg Psychiatr 1965;28:282.
14. Wang JD, Huang CC, Hwang YH, et al. Manganese induced parkinsonism: an outbreak due to an unrepaired ventilation control system in a ferromanganese smelter. Br J Ind Med 1989;46(12):856–9.
15. Huang CC, Chu NS, Lu CS, et al. Chronic manganese intoxication. Arch Neurol 1989;46(10):1104–6.
16. Huang CC, Chu NS, Lu CS, et al. Long-term progression in chronic manganism: ten years of follow-up. Neurology 1998;50(3):698–700.
17. Huang CC, Lu CS, Chu NS, et al. Progression after chronic manganese exposure. Neurology 1993;43(8):1479–83.
18. Lu CS, Huang CC, Chu NS, et al. Levodopa failure in chronic manganism [see comment]. Neurology 1994;44(9):1600–2.
19. Huang C-C, Weng Y-H, Lu C-S, et al. Dopamine transporter binding in chronic manganese intoxication. J Neurol 2003;250(11):1335–9.

20. Beintker E. The effect of manganese during arc welding. Zentralblatt Gewerbehy-giene 1932;9:207–11.
21. McMillan G. Is electric arc welding linked to manganism or Parkinson's disease? Toxicol Rev 2005;24(4):237–57.
22. Oltramare M, Tchicaloff M, Desbaumes P, et al. Chronic manganese poisoning in two arc welders. Int Arch Gewerbepathol Gewerbehyg 1965;21:124–40.
23. Nelson K, Golnick J, Korn T, et al. Manganese encephalopathy: utility of early magnetic resonance imaging. Br J Ind Med 1993;50(6):510–3.
24. Discalzi G, Pira E, Herrero Hernandez E, et al. Occupational Mn parkinsonism: magnetic resonance imaging and clinical patterns following CaNa2-EDTA chela-tion. Neurotoxicology 2000;21(5):863–6.
25. Sato K, Ueyama H, Arakawa R, et al. A case of welder presenting with parkin-sonism after chronic manganese exposure. Rinsho Shinkeigaku 2000;40(11):1110–5 [in Japanese].
26. Ono K, Komai K, Yamada M. Myoclonic involuntary movement associated with chronic manganese poisoning. J Neurol Sci 2002;199(1–2):93–6.
27. Sadek AH, Rauch R, Schulz PE. Parkinsonism due to manganism in a welder. Int J Toxicol 2003;22(5):393–401.
28. Bowler RM, Koller W, Schulz PE. Parkinsonism due to manganism in a welder: neurological and neuropsychological sequelae. Neurotoxicology 2006;27(3):327–32.
29. Kenangil G, Ertan S, Sayilir I, et al. Progressive motor syndrome in a welder with pallidal T1 hyperintensity on MRI: a two-year follow-up. Mov Disord 2006;21(12):2197–200.
30. Stobbaerts RF, Ieven M, Deelstra H, et al. Mn-content of total parenteral and enteral nutrition. Z Ernahrungswiss 1992;31(2):138–46.
31. Roels H, Meiers G, Delos M, et al. Influence of the route of administration and the chemical form (MnCl2, MnO2) on the absorption and cerebral distribution of manganese in rats. Arch Toxicol 1997;71(4):223–30.
32. Jenkins N, Eagar T. Chemical analysis of welding fume particles. Welding J 2005; 84:87s–93s.
33. Dickinson D, Lippold J. Analysis of welding fume from E6010 and E308-16 elec-trodes. Dublin (OH): D&L Welding Fume Analysis, LLC; 2004. p. 1–64.
34. Dickinson D, Lippold J. Analysis of welding fume from Lincore M Electrodes. Dublin (OH): D&L Welding Fume Analysis, LLC; 2005. p. 1–37.
35. Lippold J, Dickinson D. Analysis of welding fume from Tri-mark 771 Electrodes. Dublin (OH): D&L Welding Fume Analysis, LLC; 2005. p. 1–37.
36. Bush VJ, Moyer TP, Batts KP, et al. Essential and toxic element concentrations in fresh and formalin-fixed human autopsy tissues. Clin Chem 1995;41(2):284–94.
37. Crossgrove JS, Yokel RA. Manganese distribution across the blood-brain barrier. IV. Evidence for brain influx through store-operated calcium channels. Neurotox-icology 2005;26(3):297–307.
38. Aschner M, Guilarte TR, Schneider JS, et al. Manganese: recent advances in understanding its transport and neurotoxicity. Toxicol Appl Pharmacol 2007; 221(2):131–47.
39. Murphy VA, Wadhwani KC, Smith QR, et al. Saturable transport of manganese(II) across the rat blood-brain barrier. J Neurochem 1991;57(3):948–54.
40. Wadhwani KC, Murphy VA, Smith QR, et al. Saturable transport of manganese(II) across blood-nerve barrier of rat peripheral nerve. Am J Physiol 1992;262(2 Pt 2):R284–8.

41. Yokel RA, Crossgrove JS, Bukaveckas BL. Manganese distribution across the blood-brain barrier. II. Manganese efflux from the brain does not appear to be carrier mediated. Neurotoxicology 2003;24(1):15–22.
42. Smith D, Gwiazda R, Bowler R, et al. Biomarkers of Mn exposure in humans. Am J Ind Med 2007;50(11):801–11.
43. Mahoney JP, Small WJ. Studies on manganese. 3. The biological half-life of radio-manganese in man and factors which affect this half-life. J Clin Invest 1968;47(3):643–53.
44. Mena I, Horiuchi K, Burke K, et al. Chronic manganese poisoning. Individual susceptibility and absorption of iron. Neurology 1969;19(10):1000–6.
45. Dastur D, Manghani D, Raghavendran K. Distribution and fate of ^{54}Mn in the monkey: studies of different parts of the central nervous system and other organs. J Clin Invest 1971;50(1):9–20.
46. Newland MC, Cox C, Hamada R, et al. The clearance of manganese chloride in the primate. Fund Appl Toxicol 1987;9(2):314–28.
47. Gibbons RA, Dixon SN, Hallis K, et al. Manganese metabolism in cows and goats. Biochim Biophys Acta 1976;444(1):1–10.
48. Borg DC, Cotzias GC. Incorporation of manganese into erythrocytes as evidence for a manganese porphyrin in man. Nature 1958;182(4650):1677–8.
49. Roels H, Sarhan MJ, Hanotiau I, et al. Preclinical toxic effects of manganese in workers from a Mn salts and oxides producing plant. Sci Total Environ 1985;42(1/2):201–6.
50. Roels HA, Ortega Eslava MI, Ceulemans E, et al. Prospective study on the reversibility of neurobehavioral effects in workers exposed to manganese dioxide. Neurotoxicology 1999;20(2/3):255–71.
51. Crump KS, Rousseau P. Results from eleven years of neurological health surveillance at a manganese oxide and salt producing plant. Neurotoxicology 1999;20(2/3):273–86.
52. Racette BA, McGee-Minnich L, Moerlein SM, et al. Welding-related parkinsonism: clinical features, treatment, and pathophysiology [see comment]. Neurology 2001;56(1):8–13.
53. Racette BA, Tabbal SD, Jennings D, et al. Prevalence of parkinsonism and relationship to exposure in a large sample of Alabama welders. Neurology 2005;64(2):230–5.
54. Bowler RM, Gysens S, Diamond E, et al. Manganese exposure: neuropsychological and neurological symptoms and effects in welders. Neurotoxicology 2006;27(3):315–26.
55. Bowler RM, Roels HA, Nakagawa S, et al. Dose-effect relationships between manganese exposure and neurological, neuropsychological and pulmonary function in confined space bridge welders. Occup Environ Med 2007;64(3):167–77.
56. Bowler RM, Nakagawa S, Drezgic M, et al. Sequelae of fume exposure in confined space welding: a neurological and neuropsychological case series. Neurotoxicology 2007;28(2):298–311.
57. Zoni S, Albini E, Lucchini R. Neuropsychological testing for the assessment of manganese neurotoxicity: a review and a proposal. Am J Ind Med 2007;50(11):812–30.
58. Meyer-Baron M, Knapp G, Schäper M, et al. Performance alterations associated with occupational exposure to manganese–a meta-analysis. Neurotoxicology 2009;30(4):487–96.
59. Greiffenstein MF, Lees-Haley PR. Neuropsychological correlates of manganese exposure: a meta-analysis. J Clin Exp Neuropsychol 2007;29(2):113–26.

60. Fryzek J, Hansen J, Cohen S, et al. A cohort study of Parkinson's disease and other neurodegenerative disorders in Danish welders. J Occup Environ Med 2005;47:466–72.
61. Park RM, Schulte PA, Bowman JD, et al. Potential occupational risks for neurodegenerative diseases. Am J Ind Med 2005;48(1):63–77.
62. Fored CM, Fryzek JP, Brandt L, et al. Parkinson's disease and other basal ganglia or movement disorders in a large nationwide cohort of Swedish welders. Occup Environ Med 2006;63(2):135–40.
63. Dick F, De Palma G, Ahmadi A, et al. Environmental risk factors for Parkinson's disease and parkinsonism: the Geoparkinson study. Occup Environ Med 2007; 64(10):666–72.
64. Marsh G, Gula M. Employment as a welder and Parkinson Disease among heavy equipment manufacturing workers. J Occup Environ Med 2006;48(10):1031–46.
65. Stampfer M. Welding occupations and mortality from Parkinson's disease and other neurodegenerative diseases among United States men, 1985–1999. J Occup Environ Hyg 2009;6:267–72.
66. Baek SY, Lee MJ, Jung HS. Effect of manganese exposure on MPTP neurotoxicities. Neurotoxicology 2003;24(4–5):657–65.
67. Park RM, Bowler RM, Roels HA. Exposure-response relationship and risk assessment for cognitive deficits in early welding-induced manganism. J Occup Environ Med 2009;51(10):1125–36.
68. Buchet JP, Lauwerys R, Roels H, et al. Determination of manganese in blood and urine by flameless atomic absorption spectrophotometry. Clin Chim Acta 1976; 73(3):481–6.
69. Allain P, Mauras Y, Premel-Cabic A, et al. Effects of an EDTA infusion on the urinary elimination of several elements in healthy subjects. Br J Clin Pharmacol 1991;31(3):347–9.
70. Cranton E, Liu Z, Smith I. Urinary trace and toxic elements and minerals in untimed urine specimens relative to urine creatinine, Part I: concentrations of elements in fasting urine. Journal of Advancement in Medicine 1989;2(1):331–49.
71. Sata F, Araki S, Murata K, et al. Behavior of heavy metals in human urine and blood following calcium disodium ethylenediamine tetraacetate injection: observations in metal workers. J Toxicol Environ Health A 1998;54(3):167–78.
72. Barceloux D. Manganese. Clin Toxicol 1999;37(2):293–307.
73. Anonymous. ARUP's Laboratory Test Directory. 2011. Available at: http://www.aruplab.com/guides/ug/tests/0099265.jsp. Accessed February 14, 2011.
74. Anonymous. Mayo Medical Laboratory. Rochester (MN): Mayo Clinic; 2011. Available at: http://www.mayomedicallaboratories.com/testcatalog/Clinical+and+Interpretive/89120. Accessed February 14, 2011.
75. Anonymous. LabCorp, Laboratory Corporation of America, Test Menu 2011. Available at: https://www.labcorp.com/wps/portal/provider/testmenu/. Accessed February 14, 2011.
76. Shinotoh H, Snow BJ, Hewitt KA. MRI and PET studies of manganese-intoxicated monkeys. Neurology 1995;45(6):1199–204.
77. Uchino A, Noguchi T, Nomiyama K, et al. Manganese accumulation in the brain: MR imaging. Neuroradiology 2007;49(9):715–20.
78. Hauser RA, Zesiewicz TA, Martinez C, et al. Blood manganese correlates with brain magnetic resonance imaging changes in patients with liver disease. Can J Neurol Sci 1996;23(2):95–8.
79. Krieger D, Krieger S, Jansen O, et al. Manganese and chronic hepatic encephalopathy. Lancet 1995;346(8970):270–4.

80. Nagatomo S, Umehara F, Hanada K, et al. Manganese intoxication during total parenteral nutrition: report of two cases and review of the literature. J Neurol Sci 1999;162(1):102–5.

81. Ono J, Harada K, Kodaka R, et al. Manganese deposition in the brain during long-term total parenteral nutrition. JPEN J Parenter Enteral Nutr 1995;19(4): 310–2.

82. Selikhova M, Fedoryshyn L, Matviyenko Y, et al. Parkinsonism and dystonia caused by the illicit use of ephedrone–a longitudinal study. Mov Disord 2008; 23(15):2224–31.

83. Stepens A, Logina I, Liguts V, et al. A Parkinsonian syndrome in methcathinone users and the role of manganese. N Engl J Med 2008;358(10):1009–17.

84. Dietz MC, Ihrig A, Wrazidlo W, et al. Results of magnetic resonance imaging in long-term manganese dioxide-exposed workers. Environ Res 2001;85(1):37–40.

85. Kim Y, Kim JW, Ito K, et al. Idiopathic parkinsonism with superimposed manganese exposure: utility of positron emission tomography. Neurotoxicology 1999; 20(2–3):249–52.

86. Josephs KA, Ahlskog JE, Klos KJ, et al. Neurologic manifestations in welders with pallidal MRI T1 hyperintensity [see comment]. Neurology 2005;64(12):2033–9.

87. Neiman J, Haapaniemi HM, Hillbom M. Neurological complications of drug abuse: pathophysiological mechanisms. Eur J Neurol 2000;7(6):595–606.

88. Huang CC. Parkinsonism induced by chronic manganese intoxication–an experience in Taiwan. Chang Gung Med J 2007;30(5):385–95.

89. Huang CC, Chu NS, Lu CS, et al. The natural history of neurological manganism over 18 years. Parkinsonism Relat Disord 2007;13(3):143–5.

90. Chang Y, Woo S-T, Kim Y, et al. Pallidal index measured with three-dimensional T1-weighted gradient echo sequence is a good predictor of manganese exposure in welders. J Magn Reson Imaging 2010;31(4):1020–6.

91. Kim E, Kim Y, Cheong H-K, et al. Pallidal index on MRI as a target organ dose of manganese: structural equation model analysis. Neurotoxicology 2005;26(3): 351–9.

92. Herrero Hernandez E, Discalzi G, Valentini C, et al. Follow-up of patients affected by manganese-induced parkinsonism after treatment with CaNa2EDTA. Neurotoxicology 2006;27(3):333–9.

Neurologic Manifestations of Chronic Methamphetamine Abuse

Daniel E. Rusyniak, MD

KEYWORDS

- Methamphetamine abuse • Psychosis • Parkinson's
- Choreoathetoid • Punding • Formication

The current epidemic of methamphetamine abuse in the United States is not surprising. Methamphetamine can be produced from a wide variety of starting materials and methods. This fact is in contrast to cocaine, which is only commercially grown in South America, must be extracted from the plant, converted to its freebase form, shipped overseas (escaping detection by the Drug Enforcement Administration [DEA]), and then distributed, typically through gangs, to clients on the street.[1] Based on the attractiveness of methamphetamine to both users and its manufacturers, it is only surprising that the current outbreak of methamphetamine abuse in the United States took so long to reach epidemic proportions.

In 1893, methamphetamine was synthesized from ephedrine (derived from the plant *Ephedra sinica*) by Nagai Nagayoshi.[2,3] Eventually, a synthetic version would find its way to the consumer market as an over-the-counter (OTC) nasal decongestant and a brochodilator.[4–6] Far from an OTC drug today, the Food and Drug Administration (FDA) has characterized methamphetamine as a schedule II drug, which can only be prescribed for attention-deficit/hyperactivity disorder, extreme obesity, or to treat narcolepsy.

With the world on the brink of war, and its toxic effects not yet well described, the clinical effects of methamphetamine were thought to be ideal for the soldier in combat: increased alertness and aggression, plus decreased hunger and need to sleep. In World War II, the United States, Germany, and Japan all readily employed it with their troops[5,7]; it has been estimated that the United States alone distributed 200 million

This work was supported by USPHS grants DA020484 and DA026867.
The author has nothing to disclose.
Department of Emergency Medicine, Indiana University School of Medicine, 1050 Wishard Boulevard, Room 2200, Indianapolis, IN 46202, USA
E-mail address: drusynia@iupui.edu

Neurol Clin 29 (2011) 641–655
doi:10.1016/j.ncl.2011.05.004
0733-8619/11/$ – see front matter © 2011 Elsevier Inc. All rights reserved.

neurologic.theclinics.com

tablets to troops.[4] After the war, Japan experienced widespread abuse as army surpluses flooded the market. Although methamphetamine usage in Japan declined in the 1960s, it resurged in the 1970s and continues to be a problem today.[7,8] In 1954, at the height of its first epidemic, there were an estimated 2 million methamphetamine users in Japan. Although still highest in Asia, methamphetamine abuse has become a worldwide epidemic. A 2008 United Nations Office on Drugs and Crime Reports estimated 25 million abusers of amphetamines worldwide, exceeding the number of users for both cocaine (14 million) and heroin (11 million).[9]

After World War II, many US soldiers and civilians continued to use methamphetamine, which at that time was available by prescription in an injectable form. When Abbott and Burroughs-Wellcome withdrew their injectable formulations in the early 1960s, an opportunity arose for the illegal manufacturing and distribution of methamphetamine.[4] West Coast motorcycle gangs, such as the infamous Hells Angels, quickly seized on this opportunity, and by the 1970s gangs were largely responsible for the manufacturing, distribution, and use of methamphetamine in the United States. It was from the transportation of methamphetamine in the crankshafts of motorcycles that it got its street name of crank.[10] At that time, methamphetamine was produced primarily from the precursors phenyl-2-propanone and methylamine (the P-2-P method).[5,8] The combination of a crack down by the Department of Justice on West Coast gangs and the Controlled Substances Act of 1970, which made the ingredients of the P-2-P method controlled substances, resulted in a shift in the manufacturing and distribution of methamphetamine to small makeshift laboratories.

In the 1980s, a crystalline form of methamphetamine that could be smoked, called ice, began to be imported from Asia to Hawaii.[10] This highly addictive form of methamphetamine quickly found its way to the US West Coast and slowly began working it way east[11]; by 1990, methamphetamine had replaced cocaine as the stimulant of choice among drug users in many areas of California.[12] What would ultimately propel methamphetamine abuse to the forefront of the DEA war on drugs, and to the front pages of mainstream magazines and newspapers, was the rural meth lab. Unlike the cultivation of the coca leaf or opium poppy, the manufacture of methamphetamine is not limited by geographic location. By using OTC ephedrine and pseudoephedrine as the main precursors, making methamphetamine became simpler and more efficient. Methamphetamine laboratories manufacturing relatively pure crystal methamphetamine began to pop up across the Midwest; with the small investment of approximately $200, a methamphetamine cook could easily earn between $2000 and $5000.[13] Despite the relative simplicity of its synthesis (by traditional chemistry standards), cooking methamphetamine requires heating volatile hydrocarbons. When done by those without chemistry backgrounds and, as it often is, in poorly ventilated areas, fires and explosions can ensue. In fact, many methamphetamine laboratories have been discovered only after they have caught fire or exploded.[14,15] In an attempt to decrease the growing methamphetamine crisis, Congress passed the 2005 Combat Methamphetamine Epidemic Act, which limited access to pseudoephedrine. This limitation shut down vast numbers of small and medium-sized laboratories, resulting in a decline in the number of admissions for methamphetamine abuse in 2006—the first time in 10 years.[10]

With increasing numbers of large-scale manufacturers in Mexico, and other parts of the world, methamphetamine continues to be a significant problem in the United States. Because it has its most devastating effects on the central nervous system (CNS), it is important for neurologists to recognize signs of abuse and the many neurologic problems caused by methamphetamine. This article should help the practicing neurologist recognize and treat these patients, improving their chance to function drug free in society.

PHARMACOLOGY AND TOXICOLOGY

Both the acute and chronic neurologic effects of methamphetamine are the result of its pharmacology and toxicology. The acute effects of methamphetamine are those of the flight-or-fight response: increased heart rate and blood pressure, vasoconstriction, bronchodilation, and hyperglycemia.[16] In addition, methamphetamine causes CNS stimulation, which may result in euphoria, increased energy and alertness, intense curiosity and emotions, decreased anxiety, and enhanced self-esteem.[16]

Whether snorted, smoked, or injected, methamphetamine rapidly crosses the blood brain barrier where it can exert powerful effects on several neurochemical systems. Because of its lipophilic nature, methamphetamine has increased CNS penetration and is more potent than its parent compound, amphetamine.[17] Once in the CNS, it binds to dopamine, norepinephrine, and, to a lesser extent, serotonin transporters located on neuronal cell membranes; at higher concentrations, methamphetamine may also cross the cell membranes independent of transporter binding. Once bound, transporters pump methamphetamine into the neuron where it is taken up by vesicular monoamine transporters. The high pKa (pKa =10.1) of methamphetamine[18] disrupts the proton gradient, which normally keeps monoamines within the vesicle. This causes monamines to leave the vesicle and accumulate in the cytoplasm where they are reverse transported out of the cell through the same transporters that pumped methamphetamine into the cell.[19,20]

In addition to increasing their release, methamphetamine also decreases monoamine reuptake and enzyme degradation.[21] The net result is that methamphetamine causes a rapid and sustained increase in the extracellular concentrations of monoamines. One of the reasons methamphetamine has exceeded cocaine in worldwide usage is that it has a longer half-life (12 hours compared with 90 minutes) and, therefore, a much longer duration of action,[22] allowing the drug addict to have a longer and more sustained high. Although many receptors have been implicated in mediating the complex physiologic responses to amphetamines, the underlying clinical effects associated with methamphetamine use involve excessive stimulation of the sympathetic nervous system. It is the rapid and sustained activation of this system that is responsible for methamphetamine's recognizable adrenergic toxidrome: tachycardia, hypertension, mydriasis, diaphoresis, and psychomotor agitation. In addition, it is the prolonged release of central monoamines and activation of the sympathetic nervous system that is responsible for most of the acute neurologic complications associated with methamphetamine use (eg, strokes, seizures, agitation, and hyperthermia).[20,23,24] The sustained and repeated release of central monoamines is also largely to blame for the chronic neurologic effects of methamphetamine abuse.[20]

With repeated use in both humans and experimental animal models, methamphetamine depletes the brain's stores of dopamine and damages dopamine and serotonin nerve terminals. This may be a contributing factor to methamphetamine's high abuse potential; without the drug, users may have an impaired ability to experience pleasure (anhedonia), slipping into a deep depression. Based on current evidence, the complex mechanisms by which methamphetamine damages neurons involves increases in intracellular and extracellular concentrations of dopamine, which sets off a cascade of events, including oxidative stress, neuroinflammation, and excitatory neurotoxicity.[25]

It has also been shown that hyperthermia, a known complication of methamphetamine use, exacerbates this neurotoxicity.[25] Although this article focuses predominantly on methamphetamine, the similarities in the pharmacology, toxicology, and clinical effects between methamphetamine, amphetamine, and other stimulants (eg, cocaine and 3,4-methylenedioxmethamphemine [ecstasy]) makes the following discussions on neurologic complications largely translatable to other CNS stimulants.

NEUROPSYCHIATRIC COMPLICATIONS

Dopamine and serotonin neurons project widely throughout the CNS and are known to influence a variety of behaviors and functions. It should not be surprising that chronic methamphetamine abuse, which can damage dopamine and serotonin nerve terminals, is associated with deficits in neuropsychological testing. It has been estimated that 40% of methamphetamine users have abnormalities on neuropsychiatric tests.[26] In a well-done meta-analysis of studies examining the effects of chronic methamphetamine abuse on neuropsychiatric function, the most frequently reported deficits involve episodic memory, executive function, and motor function.[27] Of these, the greatest impairments are in episodic memory; this form of memory is thought to be the most susceptible to neuronal dysfunction.[28] As episodic memory allows one to consciously re-experience past events,[28] methamphetamine users who, by virtue of damaged episodic memory, forget past mistakes associated with their drug usage may be doomed to repeat them.

Another effect of chronic methamphetamine abuse is damage to executive function. With impaired executive function, methamphetamine abusers are likely to be distractible, impulsive, act inappropriately despite social cues to the contrary, and lack goals. In studies, patients addicted to methamphetamine prefer smaller, immediate rewards over larger, delayed rewards.[29] To overcome that wish for immediate rewards, addicts must activate the higher cognitive control systems, which, by virtue of their damaged executive system, is not an easy task for methamphetamine-dependent individuals.[29] Another consequence of impaired executive function, demonstrated in patients with damaged frontal lobes, is perseveration: the inability to change behavior even when the current behavior becomes destructive.[30] It is easy to imagine how damage to episodic memory and executive function might result in continued methamphetamine abuse despite the physical and emotional toil it reaps on users and their families. By chemically converting users into a modern Phineas Gage, methamphetamine exerts a powerful influence on behavior and decision making. Although not specifically tested, it is also possible that persons with damaged episodic memory and executive function, before using drugs, may be more susceptible to drug abuse and addiction and may have a greater risk for relapse.

Although studies show motor deficits in chronic methamphetamine abusers, these deficits do not typically involve gross movements, as with Parkinson's disease, but rather affect fine-motor dexterity (eg, placing pegs in a pegboard). These deficits would seem to be in line with studies showing that damage to dopamine terminals is more prevalent in the caudate (more involved in cognitive motor activities) then the putamen (more involved in pure motor activities) regions of the basal ganglia.[31,32]

Along with neuropsychiatric deficits, methamphetamine abusers suffer from mental illnesses, with anxiety,[33–35] depression,[27,35–37] and psychosis[22,27,37,38] being the most commonly reported. Of these, the neurologist is perhaps most likely to be confronted with patients suffering from psychosis.

After World War II, Japan suffered not only from a methamphetamine epidemic but also from an epidemic of drug-induced psychosis.[39–42] It has been estimated that at its height (between 1945–1955), there were as many as 200,000 persons in Japan with drug-induced psychosis.[42] Although much of the research on methamphetamine-induced psychosis has been conducted in Japan, similar reports have been reported in the United States and other countries.[43,44]

The symptoms of methamphetamine-induced psychosis are similar to those seen with schizophrenia; the most frequently reported symptoms are delusions of persecution and auditory hallucinations.[39–42,44–46] Although not as commonly reported, negative symptoms (eg, poverty of speech and psychomotor retardation) have also been seen with methamphetamine-induced psychosis.[44] In addition to a similar symptomatology, both schizophrenia and amphetamine-evoked psychosis can be effectively treated with dopamine antagonists.[47] The similarities between these disorders have lead many researchers to use amphetamines to model schizophrenia in laboratory animals.[42,48]

The development of psychosis is more readily seen in people using higher methamphetamine concentrations for prolonged periods of time.[39,45,46,49,50] The reported doses required, duration of abuse, and onset of symptoms are highly variable, as is the duration of psychotic symptoms (from 1 week to an indefinite duration).[16,51] Even if symptoms abate with abstinence, they can reemerge with repeat usage or under stressful situations.[40] One of the debates associated with psychosis and methamphetamine is whether it is the result of methamphetamine-induced neurotoxicity (ie, altered dopaminergic neurotransmission) or whether the 2 disorders coexist so that persons with mental illness are more likely to abuse methamphetamine (so-called dual diagnosis). The later seems to be supported by data showing that persons with predispositions to mental illness, such as strong family histories, are significantly more likely to develop methamphetamine-associated psychosis.[49,50] Furthermore, schizophrenics given low doses of methamphetamine will have exacerbations of their symptoms.[52] Therefore, it has been suggested that in susceptible individuals methamphetamine abuse may be a trigger that unmasks schizophrenia/psychosis.[53] Others have suggested that persons with schizophrenia/psychosis seek out illicit drugs as a form of self-treatment,[54] or, as recent data suggests, that neuronal deficits underlying the development of schizophrenia make individuals more prone to develop drug addiction.[55] Either way, it is clear that methamphetamine abuse can result in the development of acute and, in some cases, chronic psychosis and that practicing neurologists should be aware of this association. With the significant increase in the number of persons abusing methamphetamine, it remains to be seen if there will be a concomitant rise in patients requiring treatment for psychosis.

FORMICATION

One interesting aspect of chronic methamphetamine psychosis is the delusion of parasitosis or formication (the thought that one is infested with and being bitten by bugs).[43,46,56–59] Commonly known as *meth mites*, this is a frequent complaint in heavy daily users of methamphetamine. In studies of patients admitted to drug treatment facilities for methamphetamine abuse, approximately 40% of the patients report having had formication[43,46]; if the patients had ever suffered from psychosis, then the percentage of persons experiencing formication rose to 70%.[46] It is interesting that similar symptoms have been reported in animals chronically administered d-amphetamine.[57,58,60] These delusions may cause patients to repetitively pick at their skin resulting in scarring of their face and extremities.[59,61] Constant picking combined with neglect of hygiene also increase the risk for developing skin infections, including abscesses and cellulitis from methicillin-resistant *Staphylococcus aureus*.[62] Along with abstinence from drug usage, dopamine antagonists have been shown to help patients with drug-induced formication.[57] Although formication is not unique to methamphetamine (it has also been reported with cocaine[63] and schizophrenia[57]), the finding of multiple pockmarks on a patient's face and extremities, or recurrent skin abscesses in these areas, should increase a clinician's suspicion of chronic metham-phetamine abuse.

STEREOTYPY OR PUNDING

One of the unique manifestations of methamphetamine abuse is the development of punding. The word *punding* is Swedish for "blockhead."[64,65] It was first coined by Rylander, who learned of the slang term from chronic amphetamine and phenmetra-zine (another stimulant abused in Sweden in the 1960s) users as they described the abnormal persistent behaviors displayed by themselves and other addicts.[64] Punding has since become a term for non–goal-directed repetitive activity. Patient-reported examples include assembling and disassembling clocks and watches or incessantly sorting through purses. What makes these behaviors troublesome is the duration of time users would dedicate to such tasks without any apparent gain. There seems to be a predilection for punding to entail activities that users had previously been involved with. For example, a carpenter abusing amphetamines may repetitively build wooden objects; artists may doodle, paint, or draw excessively; a businessman may make and add to spreadsheets for hours.[66] There is also a gender-related component: men typically tinkering with electronics and women more commonly involved in grooming behaviors, such as hair brushing and nail polishing.[64,65,67–69] It is interesting that stereotyped repetitive movements, such as head bobbing, licking, gnawing, and sniffing, are also seen in a variety of animals given amphetamines.[70]

Although first reported in amphetamine abusers, punding has also been reported in cocaine users[71] and, more recently, in patients with Parkinson's disease receiving dopamine replacement therapy.[66,67] Similar to chronic stimulant abusers, patients with Parkinson's disease have dysfunctional dopaminergic neurotransmission and can develop psychosis.[67] This finding suggests a similar pathophysiologic mechanism. Although few controlled studies have been done on punding with substance abuse, there is some data available on its incidence. In a study of 50 patients addicted to cocaine, Fasano reported that 38% had some form of punding.[66] These patients spent, on average, 3 hours a day engaged in their repetitive activities.[66] One patient reported spending up to 14 hours a day playing computer games and collecting things.[67] It is interesting that the majority of interviewed patients in this study reported that their behavior began shortly after their first drug usage. In addition, the duration and amount of drug use did not seem to predict which users would develop punding and which would not.[67] This finding suggests that, like the development of stimulant-induced psychosis, there may be a predisposition for the development of punding that is merely brought out by the drug. As previously discussed, the same abnormal brain circuitry that increases one's risk for becoming addicted may also be involved in the develop-ment of such stereotyped behaviors. In his first report on the topic, Rylander described punding in 26% (40 of 150) of the amphetamine addicts he interviewed.[64] These patients shared identical symptomatology as the cocaine addicts and patients with Parkinson's disease who engaged in punding. The majority of the drug addicts did not describe associated anxiety or distress over their activities, but thought of them with amusement. Some even found them pleasurable. When abstaining from drug usage, punding typically abates. Although the neurologic mechanisms behind punding are not yet well delineated, it appears to involve dopamine. Repeated dosing of amphetamines in animals results in behavioral sensitization. This sensitization is man-ifested as increased locomotion and stereotypic behavior with each subsequent dose of amphetamine. This sensitization appears to involve both glutamate and dopamine, and, more recently, dopamine-mediated decreases in acetylcholine have been implicated.[67,72,73] As concentrations of extracellular dopamine increase with each subsequent dose of amphetamine, one could envision over time this excess dopamine causing neurotoxicity or change the normal balance between dopamine 1 (D1) and dopamine 2 (D2) receptor activity[52]; In a review on the topic, Fasano makes a strong argument for the involvement of both D1 and D2 receptors in the development of punding, and suggests that, if needed, treatments might include atypical antipsychotics.[66]

CHRONIC METHAMPHETAMINE ABUSE AND THE DEVELOPMENT OF PARKINSON'S DISEASE

People with Parkinson's disease[66,67] also exhibit unusual impulse-control disorders and punding. Similar to methamphetamine abusers, patients with Parkinson's disease, whether they are newly diagnosed[74] or have had dopamine-replacement therapies,[75] have gender-specific compulsivity problems. Men more frequently suffer from pathologic gambling and compulsive sexual behavior, whereas women tend toward compulsive buying and binge eating. The collective animal and human data clearly show that high-dose methamphetamine abuse causes alterations in striatal dopaminergic neurotransmission. Numerous pathology and imaging studies have shown reductions in striatal dopamine, tyrosine hydroxylase, and dopamine transporters.[6,32,76-80] Because these findings are also found in persons with Parkinson's disease, it is logical to expect that chronic methamphetamine addicts would develop signs of Parkinson's disease.

The current and prevailing theory is that abusing methamphetamine does not increase one's risk of developing Parkinson's disease or Parkinsonism.[31,32,76] Several hypotheses have been put forth to explain the discrepancy between the research and clinical data.[31,32,76] The simplest hypothesis is that they are different disorders. Parkinson's disease involves loss of dopaminergic neurons in the substantia nigra, whereas methamphetamine abuse causes alterations in dopaminergic nerve terminals, but not in the cell bodies themselves.[32] In studies of methamphetamine abusers, the reductions in dopamine have a different distribution than in patients with Parkinson's disease. Methamphetamine users have greater dopamine reductions in the caudate compared with the putamen, with patients with Parkinson's disease showing the opposite.[32] Another hypothesis is that once users become drug abstinent, the damaged dopaminergic nerve terminals begin to recover; decreases in dopamine transporters of methamphetamine abusers were found to significantly recover with prolonged (>12 months) abstinence.[79]

Another hypothesis is that methamphetamine abusers do not actually damage their dopaminergic nerve terminals, and that the findings of reduce dopamine levels represent a compensatory response to repeated elevations in monoamines. The strongest argument for this has been that the vesicular transporter-2 (VMAT2), which is known to be reduced in Parkinson's disease and to be resistant to drug-compensatory regulation, is not significantly reduced in abstinent methamphetamine abusers.[6,81] In fact, a more recent positron emission tomography (PET) study of nonabstinent methamphetamine abusers found increases in VMAT2.[82] This finding was thought to be caused by reductions in vesicular dopamine, depleted from recent release, resulting in less dopamine being available to compete for binding to VMAT2.[82]

Another intriguing hypothesis involves nicotine and nicotine receptors. Acetylcholine nicotinic mechanisms can influence the behavioral and neurochemical effects of psychomotor stimulant drugs and vice versa.[83] An overwhelming number of methamphetamine users smoke cigarettes compared with the general population (87%–92% vs 22%).[84] Because cigarette smoking negatively correlates with development of Parkinson's disease,[85] methamphetamine abusers may be protected or self-treated.[31]

Some researchers think that methamphetamine abuse does increase the risk for developing Parkinson's disease.[76,86,87] One retrospective study, looking at hospital admissions over a 10-year period, found an increased incidence of Parkinson's disease among patients who had a prior history of being admitted with a methamphetamine-related problem.[87] Because it may take many years before reductions in dopamine reach the levels mediating clinical symptoms, it is possible that the patients enrolled in many of the prospective clinical studies are not old enough to show symptoms; the majority of studies involve young adults. What instead may occur is that as methamphetamine use increases in young adults, we may see a shift in the age of onset of Parkinson's disease. There have been 2 studies involving the same group of patients that support this idea. In a phone survey of patients with Parkinson's disease receiving care at 1 of 3 clinics, patients with Parkinson's disease were significantly more likely (odds ratio = 8, confidence interval 1.6–41.4) to have used amphetamines than their unaffected spouses,[88] and in the majority of these patients, their exposures to amphetamines occurred years (~27) before symptoms onset.[88] Compared with patients with Parkinson's disease without a history of exposure, those patients with a history of amphetamine use were significantly younger at the age of symptom onset, but not at the age of diagnosis.[86] This study is small, however, and subject, by its design, to recall bias. Further work is needed to confirm whether there is, in fact, an association between amphetamine use and the development of Parkinson's disease.

CHOREOATHETOID MOVEMENTS AND DYSKINESIAS

A potential complication of methamphetamine-induced damage to the dopaminergic nervous system is the development of dyskinesias and choreoathetoid movements.[89] There have been numerous reports of choreoathetoid movements (involuntary purposeless and uncontrollable movements with features of both chorea and athetosis) in patients using or abusing amphetamines.[46,68,69,90–94] In one report, patients with underlying chorea (Sydenham, Huntington, and Lupus) were given an intravenous dose of amphetamine to assess its effect on their baseline movements. In each of these patients, amphetamine dramatically worsened their underlying chorea.[95] The increases in limb movements provoked by amphetamines could be prevented if patients were pretreated with the D2 antagonist haloperidol.[95] Because a group of control patients without chorea that were given amphetamine did not develop movement disorders, the investigators suggested that the development of chorea from amphetamines may require a underlying damage to the striatum.[95] This supposition would seem to be supported from several lines of evidence. For one, numerous studies have shown that methamphetamine abusers have evidence of dopaminergic neurotoxicity in the striatum.[6,25,96] Additionally, chronic methamphetamine abusers, even without frank chorea, often have demonstrable movement disorders.[97] Furthermore, in some patients, movement disorders can last for years even after they have stopped using amphetamines.[64,68] Lastly, patients who have stopped abusing amphetamine, and subsequently recovered from their choreoathetoid movement disorder, will often redevelop symptoms the first time they use amphetamines again, suggesting that patients may become permanently susceptible.[68]

The description of choreoathetoid movements typically involves the limbs, neck, and face and often has a rhythmic dancelike quality. Similar to other dyskinesias, symptoms disappear while patients sleep.[68] Although in some patients dopamine antagonists and benzodiazepines have been found to relieve symptoms,[69,91,95] in others they have had no benefit.[68] Not limited to amphetamines, choreoathetoid movements have also been reported with other stimulants, including cocaine (known as crack dancing).[64,97–99] Although the paucity of literature on this topic suggests that the development of these symptoms is rare, the fact that there are street names for this in English and Spanish suggests that it may occur more commonly than reported.[98] It is a sad and real possibility that, among other reasons, many of the homeless persons seen dancing and writhing around on the street corners of many major cities may be manifesting signs of stimulant-induced choreoathetoid movements.

DENTAL CARIES

Although not traditionally considered a neurologic complication, the development of dental caries and teeth erosion in chronic methamphetamine abusers may be the result of elevations in brain monoamines. Referred to as *meth mouth*, advanced dental caries, tooth loss, and tooth fractures seen among methamphetamine users is the result of decreased saliva production (xerostomia) combined with teeth grinding (bruxism) and jaw clenching.[100–108] Additional contributors to methamphetamine-related tooth decay include poor oral hygiene combined with the consumption of sugar-containing carbonated soft drinks, which is a common habit among methamphetamine users, with Mountain Dew being their drink of choice.[100–102,106,109] Dental caries seen with meth mouth occur in a similar pattern to other disorders involving xerostomia (eg, Sjögren and radiation), involving the buccal smooth surface of the posterior teeth and the interproximal areas of the anterior teeth.[100,102] Decay can progress to complete destruction of dental enamel, with many young methamphetamine addicts requiring dentures.[110] The mechanism of methamphetamine-induced xerostomia appears to be mediated by central alpha-2 receptors, which, when bound by norepinephrine, decreases salivary flow.[103,109,111] Along with increasing dopamine, methamphetamine causes sustained increases in extracellular concentrations of norepinephrine.[112] Although the cause of bruxism is not well known, it is thought to be of central origin and, likewise, to involve central monoamines.[107,108,113] Unlike nocturnal bruxism, methamphetamine users will often have bruxism day and night.[107,108] Although the practicing neurologist is unlikely to be consulted to see patients because of dental caries, recognizing the dental and dermatologic manifestations of chronic methamphetamine abuse may help to identify at-risk patients.

SUMMARY

Chronic methamphetamine abuse has devastating effects on the CNS. The degree to which addicts will tolerate the dysfunction in the way they think, feel, move, and even look, is a powerful testimony to the addictive properties of this drug. Although the mechanisms behind these disorders are complex, at their heart they involve the recurring increase in the concentrations of central monoamines with subsequent dysfunction in dopaminergic neurotransmission. The mainstay of treatment for the problems associated with chronic methamphetamine abuse is abstinence. However, by recognizing the manifestations of chronic abuse, clinicians will be better able to help their patients get treatment for their addiction and to deal with the neurologic complications related to chronic abuse.

ACKNOWLEDGMENTS

The author would like to acknowledge the valuable editorial assistance of Pamela J. Durant.

REFERENCES

1. Streatfeild D. Cocaine: an unauthorized biography. New York: Picador; 2001.
2. Nagai T, Kamiyama S. Forensic toxicologic analysis of methamphetamine and amphetamine optical isomers by high performance liquid chromatography. Int J Legal Med 1988;101:151–9.
3. Nagai H. Studies on the components of *Ephedraceae* in herb medicine. Yahugaku Zasshi 1893;139:901–33.
4. Miller MA. History and epidemiology of amphetamine abuse in the United States. In: Klee H, editor. Amphetamine misuse: international perspectives on current trends. Reading (UK): Harwood Academic Publishers; 1997. p. 113–33.
5. Anglin MD, Burke C, Perrochet B, et al. History of the methamphetamine problem. J Psychoactive Drugs 2000;32:137–41.
6. Wilson JM, Kalasinsky KS, Levey AI, et al. Striatal dopamine nerve terminal markers in human, chronic methamphetamine users. Nat Med 1996;2:699–703.
7. Suwaki H, Fukui S, Konuma K. Methamphetamine abuse in Japan: its 45 year history and the current situation. In: Klee H, editor. Amphetamine misuse: international perspectives on current trends. Reading (UK): Harwood Academic Publishers; 1997.
8. Hunt D, Kuck S, Truitt L. Methamphetamine use: lessons learned: report to the National Institute of Justice. Cambridge (MA): Abt Associates Inc; 2006. Available at: http://www.ncjrs.gov/pdffiles1/nij/grants/209730.pdf. Accessed May 10, 2011.
9. UNDOC. Annual Report 2008. 2008. Available at: www.unodc.org/documents/about-unodc/AR08_WEB.pdf. Accessed January 19, 2011.
10. Gonzales R, Mooney L, Rawson RA. The Methamphetamine Problem in the United States. Annu Rev Public Health 2010;31:385–98.
11. Office of National Drug Control Policy. II. America's Drug Use Profile. Available at: http://www.ncjrs.gov/ondcppubs/publications/policy/ndcs01/chap2.html. Accessed January 19, 2011.
12. Derlet RW, Heischober B. Methamphetamine. Stimulant of the 1990s? West J Med 1990;153:625–8.
13. Costs of Meth. Available at: http://www5.semo.edu/criminal/medfels/text_meth_cost.htm. Accessed January 19, 2011.
14. Denehy J. The meth epidemic: its effect on children and communities. J Sch Nurs 2006;22:63–5.
15. Betsinger G. Coping with meth lab hazards. Occup Health Saf 2006;75:50, 52, 54–8, passim.
16. Cruickshank CC, Dyer KR. A review of the clinical pharmacology of methamphetamine. Addiction 2009;104:1085–99.
17. Lake CR, Quirk RS. CNS stimulants and look-alike drugs. Psychiatr Clin North Am 1984;7:689–701.
18. Brandle E, Fritzsch G, Greven J. Affinity of different local anesthetic drugs and catecholamines for the contraluminal transport system for organic cations in proximal tubules of rat kidneys. J Pharmacol Exp Ther 1992;260:734–41.
19. Fleckenstein AE, Volz TJ, Riddle EL, et al. New insights into the mechanism of action of amphetamines. Annu Rev Pharmacol Toxicol 2007;47:681–98.
20. Schep LJ, Slaughter RJ, Beasley DM. The clinical toxicology of metamfetamine. Clin Toxicol (Phila) 2010;48:675–94.
21. Suzuki O, Hattori H, Asano M, et al. Inhibition of monoamine oxidase by d-methamphetamine. Biochem Pharmacol 1980;29:2071–3.

22. Meredith CW, Jaffe C, Ang-Lee K, et al. Implications of chronic methamphetamine use: a literature review. Harv Rev Psychiatry 2005;13:141–54.
23. O'Connor AD, Rusyniak DE, Bruno A. Cerebrovascular and cardiovascular complications of alcohol and sympathomimetic drug abuse. Med Clin North Am 2005;89:1343–58.
24. Rusyniak DE, Sprague JE. Hyperthermic syndromes induced by toxins. Clin Lab Med 2006;26:165–84.
25. Yamamoto BK, Moszczynska A, Gudelsky GA. Amphetamine toxicities. Ann N Y Acad Sci 2010;1187:101–21.
26. Rippeth JD, Heaton RK, Carey CL, et al. Methamphetamine dependence increases risk of neuropsychological impairment in HIV infected persons. J Int Neuropsychol Soc 2004;10:1–14.
27. Scott JC, Woods SP, Matt GE, et al. Neurocognitive effects of methamphetamine: a critical review and meta-analysis. Neuropsychol Rev 2007;17:275–97.
28. Tulving E. Episodic memory: from mind to brain. Annu Rev Psychol 2002;53:1–25.
29. Hoffman WF, Schwartz DL, Huckans MS, et al. Cortical activation during delay discounting in abstinent methamphetamine dependent individuals. Psychopharmacology (Berl) 2008;201:183–93.
30. Gilbert SJ, Burgess PW. Executive function. Curr Biol 2008;18:R110–4.
31. Caligiuri MP, Buitenhuys C. Do preclinical findings of methamphetamine-induced motor abnormalities translate to an observable clinical phenotype? Neuropsychopharmacology 2005;30:2125–34.
32. Moszczynska A, Fitzmaurice P, Ang L, et al. Why is parkinsonism not a feature of human methamphetamine users? Brain 2004;127(Pt 2):363–70.
33. Glasner-Edwards S, Mooney LJ, Marinelli-Casey P, et al. Anxiety disorders among methamphetamine dependent adults: association with post-treatment functioning. Am J Addict 2010;19:385–90.
34. Hall W, Hando J, Darke S, et al. Psychological morbidity and route of administration among amphetamine users in Sydney, Australia. Addiction 1996;91:81–7.
35. McKetin R, Ross J, Kelly E, et al. Characteristics and harms associated with injecting versus smoking methamphetamine among methamphetamine treatment entrants. Drug Alcohol Rev 2008;27:277–85.
36. Copeland AL, Sorensen JL. Differences between methamphetamine users and cocaine users in treatment. Drug Alcohol Depend 2001;62:91–5.
37. Newton TF, Kalechstein AD, Duran S, et al. Methamphetamine abstinence syndrome: preliminary findings. Am J Addict 2004;13:248–55.
38. Nordahl TE, Salo R, Leamon M. Neuropsychological effects of chronic methamphetamine use on neurotransmitters and cognition: a review. J Neuropsychiatry Clin Neurosci 2003;15:317–35.
39. Iwanami A, Sugiyama A, Kuroki N, et al. Patients with methamphetamine psychosis admitted to a psychiatric hospital in Japan. A preliminary report. Acta Psychiatr Scand 1994;89:428–32.
40. Sato M. A lasting vulnerability to psychosis in patients with previous methamphetamine psychosis. Ann N Y Acad Sci 1992;654:160–70.
41. Shimazono Y, Matsushima E. Behavioral and neuroimaging studies on schizophrenia in Japan. Psychiatry Clin Neurosci 1995;49:3–11.
42. Yui K, Ikemoto S, Ishiguro T, et al. Studies of amphetamine or methamphetamine psychosis in Japan: relation of methamphetamine psychosis to schizophrenia. Ann N Y Acad Sci 2000;914:1–12.
43. Hawks D, Mitcheson M, Ogborne A, et al. Abuse of methylamphetamine. Br Med J 1969;2:715–21.

44. Srisurapanont M, Ali R, Marsden J, et al. Psychotic symptoms in methamphetamine psychotic in-patients. Int J Neuropsychopharmacol 2003;6:347–52.
45. Mahoney JJ 3rd, Kalechstein AD, De La Garza R 2nd, et al. Presence and persistence of psychotic symptoms in cocaine- versus methamphetamine-dependent participants. Am J Addict 2008;17:83–98.
46. Ellinwood EH. Amphetamine Psychosis: I. Description of the individuals and process. J Nerv Ment Dis 1967;144:273–83.
47. Angrist B, Lee HK, Gershon S. The antagonism of amphetamine-induced symptomatology by a neuroleptic. Am J Psychiatry 1974;131:817–9.
48. Snyder SH. Amphetamine psychosis: a "model" schizophrenia mediated by catecholamines. Am J Psychiatry 1973;130:61–7.
49. Chen CK, Lin SK, Sham PC, et al. Pre-morbid characteristics and co-morbidity of methamphetamine users with and without psychosis. Psychol Med 2003;33: 1407–14.
50. Chen CK, Lin SK, Sham PC, et al. Morbid risk for psychiatric disorder among the relatives of methamphetamine users with and without psychosis. Am J Med Genet 2005;136B:87–91.
51. Bell DS. The experimental reproduction of amphetamine psychosis. Arch Gen Psychiatry 1973;29:35–40.
52. Lieberman JA, Kinon BJ, Loebel AD. Dopaminergic mechanisms in idiopathic and drug-induced psychoses. Schizophr Bull 1990;16:97–110.
53. Bell DS. Comparison of amphetamine psychosis and schizophrenia. Br J Psychiatry 1965;111:701–7.
54. Buckley PF. Substance abuse in schizophrenia: a review. J Clin Psychiatry 1998; 59(Suppl 3):26–30.
55. Chambers RA, Krystal JH, Self DW. A neurobiological basis for substance abuse comorbidity in schizophrenia. Biol Psychiatry 2001;50:71–83.
56. Richards JR, Bretz SW, Johnson EB, et al. Methamphetamine abuse and emergency department utilization. West J Med 1999;170:198–202.
57. de Leon J, Antelo RE, Simpson G. Delusion of parasitosis or chronic tactile hallucinosis: hypothesis about their brain physiopathology. Compr Psychiatry 1992; 33:25–33.
58. Ellinwood EH, Sudilovsky A. Chronic amphetamine intoxication: behavioral model of psychoses. In: Cole JO, Freedman AM, Friedhoff AJ, editors. Psychopathology and psychopharmacology. Baltimore (MD): Johns Hopkins University Press; 1972. p. 51–70.
59. Yaffee HS. Cutaneous stigmas associated with Methedrine (methamphetamine). Arch Dermatol 1971;104:687.
60. Ellison GD, Eison MS. Continuous amphetamine intoxication: an animal model of the acute psychotic episode. Psychol Med 1983;13:751–61.
61. Liu SW, Lien MH, Fenske NA. The effects of alcohol and drug abuse on the skin. Clin Dermatol 2010;28:391–9.
62. Cohen AL, Shuler C, McAllister S, et al. Methamphetamine use and methicillin-resistant Staphylococcus aureus skin infections. Emerg Infect Dis 2007;13: 1707–13.
63. Siegel RK. Cocaine hallucinations. Am J Psychiatry 1978;135:309–14.
64. Rylander G. Psychoses and the punding and choreiform syndromes in addiction to central stimulant drugs. Psychiatr Neurol Neurochir 1972;75: 203–12.
65. Schiorring E. Psychopathology induced by "speed drugs". Pharmacol Biochem Behav 1981;14(Suppl 1):109–22.

66. Fasano A, Petrovic I. Insights into pathophysiology of punding reveal possible treatment strategies. Mol Psychiatry 2010;15:560–73.
67. O'Sullivan SS, Evans AH, Lees AJ. Dopamine dysregulation syndrome: an overview of its epidemiology, mechanisms and management. CNS Drugs 2009;23:157–70.
68. Lundh H, Tunving K. An extrapyramidal choreiform syndrome caused by amphetamine addiction. J Neurol Neurosurg Psychiatry 1981;44:728–30.
69. Rhee KJ, Albertson TE, Douglas JC. Choreoathetoid disorder associated with amphetamine-like drugs. Am J Emerg Med 1988;6:131–3.
70. Randrup A, Munkvad I. Stereotyped activities produced by amphetamine in several animal species and man. Psychopharmacologia 1967;11:300–10.
71. Fasano A, Barra A, Nicosia P, et al. Cocaine addiction: from habits to stereotypical-repetitive behaviors and punding. Drug Alcohol Depend 2008;96:178–82.
72. Aliane V, Perez S, Bohren Y, et al. Key role of striatal cholinergic interneurons in processes leading to arrest of motor stereotypies. Brain 2010;134:110–8.
73. Pierce RC, Kalivas PW. A circuitry model of the expression of behavioral sensitization to amphetamine-like psychostimulants. Brain Res Brain Res Rev 1997;25:192–216.
74. Antonini A, Siri C, Santangelo G, et al. Impulsivity and compulsivity in drug-naive patients with Parkinson's disease. Mov Disord 2011;26:464–8.
75. Weintraub D, Koester J, Potenza MN, et al. Impulse control disorders in Parkinson disease: a cross-sectional study of 3090 patients. Arch Neurol 2010;67:589–95.
76. Guilarte TR. Is methamphetamine abuse a risk factor in parkinsonism? Neurotoxicology 2001;22:725–31.
77. McCann UD, Kuwabara H, Kumar A, et al. Persistent cognitive and dopamine transporter deficits in abstinent methamphetamine users. Synapse 2008;62:91–100.
78. Truong JG. Age-dependent methamphetamine-induced alterations in vesicular monoamine transporter-2 function: implications for neurotoxicity. J Pharmacol Exp Ther 2005;314:1087–92.
79. Volkow ND, Chang L, Wang GJ, et al. Loss of dopamine transporters in methamphetamine abusers recovers with protracted abstinence. J Neurosci 2001;21:9414–8.
80. Volkow ND, Chang L, Wang GJ, et al. Association of dopamine transporter reduction with psychomotor impairment in methamphetamine abusers. Am J Psychiatry 2001;158:377–82.
81. Johanson CE, Frey KA, Lundahl LH, et al. Cognitive function and nigrostriatal markers in abstinent methamphetamine abusers. Psychopharmacology (Berl) 2006;185:327–38.
82. Boileau I, Rusjan P, Houle S, et al. Increased vesicular monoamine transporter binding during early abstinence in human methamphetamine users: is VMAT2 a stable dopamine neuron biomarker? J Neurosci 2008;28:9850–6.
83. Desai RI, Bergman J. Drug discrimination in methamphetamine-trained rats: effects of cholinergic nicotinic compounds. J Pharmacol Exp Ther 2010;335:807–16.
84. Weinberger AH, Sofuoglu M. The impact of cigarette smoking on stimulant addiction. Am J Drug Alcohol Abuse 2009;35:12–7.
85. Hernán MA, Takkouche B, Caamaño-Isorna F, et al. A meta-analysis of coffee drinking, cigarette smoking, and the risk of Parkinson's disease. Ann Neurol 2002;52:276–84.

86. Christine CW, Garwood ER, Schrock LE, et al. Parkinsonism in patients with a history of amphetamine exposure. Mov Disord 2010;25:228–31.
87. Callaghan RC, Cunningham JK, Sajeev G, et al. Incidence of Parkinson's disease among hospital patients with methamphetamine-use disorders. Mov Disord 2010;25:2333–9.
88. Garwood ER, Bekele W, McCulloch CE, et al. Amphetamine exposure is elevated in Parkinson's disease. Neurotoxicology 2006;27:1003–6.
89. Janavs JL, Aminoff MJ. Dystonia and chorea in acquired systemic disorders. J Neurol Neurosurg Psychiatry 1998;65:436–45.
90. Shanson B. Amphetamine poisoning. Br Med J 1956;1(4966):576.
91. Downes MA, Whyte IM. Amphetamine-induced movement disorder. Emerg Med Australas 2005;17:277–80.
92. Mattson RH, Calverley JR. Dextroamphetamine-sulfate-induced dyskinesias. JAMA 1968;204:400–2.
93. Morgan JC, Winter WC, Wooten GF. Amphetamine-induced chorea in attention deficit-hyperactivity disorder. Mov Disord 2004;19:840–2.
94. Sperling LS, Horowitz JL. Methamphetamine-induced choreoathetosis and rhabdomyolysis. Ann Intern Med 1994;121:986.
95. Klawans HL, Weiner WJ. The effect of d-amphetamine on choreiform movement disorders. Neurology 1974;24:312–8.
96. Volkow ND, Chang L, Wang GJ, et al. Low level of brain dopamine D2 receptors in methamphetamine abusers: association with metabolism in the orbitofrontal cortex. Am J Psychiatry 2001;158:2015–21.
97. Bartzokis G, Beckson M, Wirshing DA, et al. Choreoathetoid movements in cocaine dependence. Biol Psychiatry 1999;45:1630–5.
98. Daras M, Koppel BS, Atos-Radzion E. Cocaine-induced choreoathetoid movements ('crack dancing'). Neurology 1994;44:751–2.
99. Stork CM, Cantor R. Pemoline induced acute choreoathetosis: case report and review of the literature. J Toxicol Clin Toxicol 1997;35:105–8.
100. Klasser GD, Epstein J. Methamphetamine and its impact on dental care. J Can Dent Assoc 2005;71:759–62.
101. ADA. Methamphetamine use and oral health. J Am Dent Assoc 2005;136:1491.
102. Shaner JW, Kimmes N, Saini T, et al. "Meth mouth": rampant caries in methamphetamine abusers. AIDS Patient Care STDS 2006;20:146–50.
103. Saini T, Edwards PC, Kimmes NS, et al. Etiology of xerostomia and dental caries among methamphetamine abusers. Oral Health Prev Dent 2005;3:189–95.
104. Donaldson M, Goodchild JH. Oral health of the methamphetamine abuser. Am J Health Syst Pharm 2006;63:2078–82.
105. Richards JR, Brofeldt BT. Patterns of tooth wear associated with methamphetamine use. J Periodontol 2000;71:1371–4.
106. Morio KA, Marshall TA, Qian F, et al. Comparing diet, oral hygiene and caries status of adult methamphetamine users and nonusers: a pilot study. J Am Dent Assoc 2008;139:171–6.
107. Winocur E, Gavish A, Voikovitch M, et al. Drugs and bruxism: a critical review. J Orofac Pain 2003;17:99–111.
108. Winocur E, Gavish A, Volfin G, et al. Oral motor parafunctions among heavy drug addicts and their effects on signs and symptoms of temporomandibular disorders. J Orofac Pain 2001;15:56–63.
109. Di Cugno F, Perec CJ, Tocci AA. Salivary secretion and dental caries experience in drug addicts. Arch Oral Biol 1981;26:363–7.

110. Shetty V, Mooney LJ, Zigler CM, et al. The relationship between methamphetamine use and increased dental disease. J Am Dent Assoc 2010;141:307–18.
111. Götrick B, Giglio D, Tobin G. Effects of amphetamine on salivary secretion. Eur J Oral Sci 2009;117:218–23.
112. Kuczenski R, Segal DS, Cho AK, et al. Hippocampus norepinephrine, caudate dopamine and serotonin, and behavioral responses to the stereoisomers of amphetamine and methamphetamine. J Neurosci 1995;15:1308–17.
113. Lobbezoo F, Naeije M. Bruxism is mainly regulated centrally, not peripherally. J Oral Rehabil 2001;28:1085–91.

Trichloroethylene and Parkinson Disease

Fariha Zaheer, MD[a], John T. Slevin, MD, MBA[a,b,c,]*

KEYWORDS

- Trichloroethylene • Idiopathic Parkinson disease
- Mitochondria • Alpha synuclein • Animal models

Idiopathic Parkinson disease (iPD) is one of the most common neurodegenerative disorders. While the incidence of iPD rises rapidly after 50 years of age,[1] it has been reported in younger age groups. The exact etiology of iPD is unknown, although both genetic and environmental agents have been implicated.[2] Multiple susceptibility genes have been discovered, and currently genetic factors are considered as the most likely cause of young-onset Parkinson disease. In case–control and cross-sectional studies, various factors have been associated with iPD including nutritional intake, living conditions, smoking, farming, and occupational chemical exposures.[3–5]

The best known chemical exposure leading to iPD is 1-methyl-4-phenyl-1,2,3,6-tetra-hydropyridine (MPTP) (**Fig. 1**). It induces clinical, pathologic and biochemical changes similar to iPD.[6] Other chemicals associated with the possible development of iPD include various pesticides,[7] industrial exposures including wood pulp and paper,[8] and various metals (eg, copper, iron, manganese, and lead).[9] Diverse mechanisms have been proposed for the development of Parkinson disease secondary to chemical exposure. The final pathway for all of these is mitochondrial oxidative stress that induces neurodegeneration predominantly involving substantia nigra.[10]

It has become clear over the last decade that iPD is a synucleinopathy. Alpha synuclein is a major component of Lewy bodies and Lewy neurites, the intraneuronal

This work was supported by the Department of Veterans Affairs Dr Slevin serves/has served on speakers' bureaus for Boehringer Ingelheim, Novartis, and Teva Pharmaceutical Industries Limited, and receives research support from Solvay Pharmaceuticals, Incorporated/Abbott, the US Department of Veterans Affairs, and the National Institutes of Health.

[a] Movement Disorders Program, Department of Neurology, University of Kentucky College of Medicine, Kentucky Clinic L-445, 740 South Limestone Street, Lexington, KY 40536-0284, USA
[b] Parkinson's Disease Consortium Center, Lexington VA Medical Center, 127-CDD, 1101 Veterans Drive, Lexington, KY 40502, USA
[c] Department of Molecular and Biomedical Pharmacology, University of Kentucky College of Medicine, Kentucky Clinic L-445, 740 South Limestone Street, Lexington, KY 40536-0284, USA
* Corresponding author. University of Kentucky College of Medicine, Kentucky Clinic L-445, 740 South Limestone Street, Lexington, KY 40536-0284.
E-mail address: jslevin@uky.edu

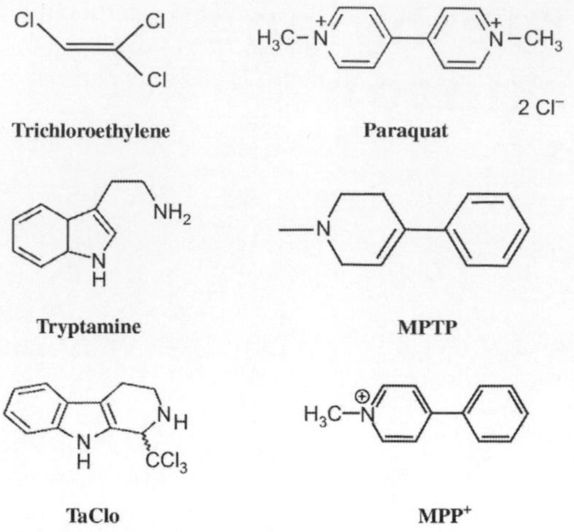

Fig. 1. Selected chemical structures.

deposits typically seen in autopsies of patients. Synuclein pathology is likely to underlie the development of clinical manifestations ranging from olfactory dysfunction to motor abnormalities and cognitive dysfunction.[11] Multiple in vivo experiments reveal that neuronal alpha synuclein is upregulated after exposure to different toxins. For example, repeated exposures of mice to the herbicide paraquat results in increased neuronal levels of synuclein.[12] A single injection of MPTP in squirrel monkeys resulted in upregulation of alpha synuclein. It has been proposed that repeated MPTP exposure leads to not only synuclein pathology but also to accelerated neurodegeneration.[13]

MITOCHONDRIAL DYSFUNCTION IN TOXIN-INDUCED PARKINSONISM

Increasing evidence suggests mitrochondrial dysfunction as a possible pathogenetic mechanism underlying the development and progression of iPD.[14] Certainly, it is the case that specific agents cause parkinsonism by their action as a mitochondrial toxin. The most well known and extensively studied agent of this class is MPTP. After systemic uptake, it is bioconverted by astrocytic monoamine oxidase type B (MAO B) to 1-methyl-4,5-phenylpyridinium (MPP$^+$). This active metabolite concentrates in dopaminergic neurons, via high-affinity dopamine transporters (DAT), where it inhibits mitochondrial complex 1 and causes cell death.[6] Reported by Langston and colleagues,[15] MPTP generated parkinsonism in a group of drug abusers after self-administration. Similarly, the pesticide rotenone, which also causes inhibition of mitochondrial complex 1, produces a clinical phenotype with biochemical and pathologic manifestations of iPD.[16] Multiple models have been developed in an attempt to define the nature and extent of mitochondrial dysfunction in association with neurotoxin-induced parkinsonism.[17] Some studies reported that mitochondrial dysfunction is limited to substantia nigra, while others indicated that it is more global in patients with iPD.[18–20] Oxidative modulation of mitochondrial proteases has been suggested as one of the mechanisms leading to mitochondrial dysfunction. Mitochondrial morphologic alterations have been reported in MPTP-exposed animals[21–23] and in hybrid cell lines populated with mitochondria from iPD patients.[24] Acute exposure of human α-synuclein transgenic mice to MPTP causes swelling of mitochondria and distortion of cristae, while chronic exposure leads to enlarged mitochondria and intra-mitochondrial inclusions.[25] Perturbation of mitochondrial calcium buffering in neurons has been observed in MPP^+-exposed mice. Alterations in autophagy and mitophagy are observed in MPTP and rotenone models as well as in genetic models of iPD.[26]

TRICHLOROETHYLENE EXPOSURE

There have been multiple reports that solvent exposure predisposes individuals to parkinsonism, but with the variety of solvents used in everyday life and in disparate occupations, solvents ranging from cleaning solutions to paints and fuels, it has been difficult to establish a clear relationship.[27,28] Among these solvents, trichloroethylene (TCE) has gained interest recently as a possible risk factor for iPD among those chronically exposed.

TCE is a chlorinated hydrocarbon whose use dates back to the 1920s. It was once used as an extractant in food processing and in anesthetic and analgesic agents. In 1977, its use for medical and food processing purposes was banned in United States.[29] It is used now as a solvent in the industrial degreasing of metals. It is also used as a secondary solvent in adhesive paint and polyvinyl chloride production. TCE is used as a solvent in the textile industry and as a solvent for adhesives and lubricants. It also has been implemented in the manufacturing of pesticides and other chemicals.[30] A nonflammable liquid with a sweet smell, it is highly lipid-soluble with a half life in adipose tissue of 5 hours. It easily penetrates into the central nervous system, and due to high lipid solubility, it slowly induces anesthesia. Cranial nerve palsies lasting for months were reported when TCE was used for anesthesia.

In recent years, TCE contamination of drinking water has become a major concern. It enters into surface waters via improper disposal and groundwater through leaks from disposal operations.[31] TCE, which can persist in water for prolonged periods, is detected in up to 30% of US drinking supplies but is within the Environmental Protection Agency's established maximum contaminant level of 0.005 mg/L.[32] It is also detected in air, soil, and food. It may enter the human body via inhalation, ingestion, or through skin.[33]

TCE is metabolized by cytochrome P450 to a trichloroethylene oxide intermediate that is converted to chloral.[34] Chloral is considered one of the precursors of 1-trichloro-methyl-1,2,3,4-tetrahydro-β-carboline, also known as TaClo,[35,36] which is readily formed under physiologic conditions from the biogenic amine tryptamine and chloral.[34] Its structural similarity to MPTP has prompted its consideration as a causative mechanism in iPD.[37] TaClo is cytotoxic when directly applied to primary cultures of dopaminergic neurons.[38,39] Significant declines in neuronal density and number[40] and dopamine turnover[41] have been reported following stereotaxic administration of TaClo into rat substantia nigra pars compacta; however, demonstrating Parkinson-like behavior has been more difficult to ascertain.[42] Although TaClo more readily crosses the blood–brain barrier than MPTP as it is more lipophilic,[43] MPP^+ is more readily and specifically concentrated in dopamine neurons by the DAT than TaClo,[44,45] perhaps explaining the greater and more immediate dopamine neuronal toxicity of exposure to MPTP. TaClo is clearly a mitochondrial toxin that can induce apoptosis through oxidative stress, mitochondrial dysfunction, and induction of apoptotic enzymes.[46] TaClo specifically inhibits electron transfer from complex 1 to ubiquinone in both rat brain homogenates and in rat liver submitochondrial particle preparations, and its potency to do so is an order of magnitude greater than that of MPP^+.[39,47]

Among multiple animal toxicity studies, until recently (see Animal Studies section) few systematically examined for central nervous system changes after chronic exposure.[29] Haglid and colleagues[48] exposed gerbils to continuous TCE for 3 months and then kept them in a TCE-free environment for 4 months to determine restoration of neurologic function. Variable effects were noted with different levels of exposure, including neuronal shrinkage, axonal swelling, and astroglial mitosis, but these generally occurred in a dose-dependent manner.[48] Briving and colleagues[49] reported increased hippocampal glutathione and dose-dependent increased high-affinity glutamate and GABA uptake in cerebellum of gerbils following 12 months of inhalation exposure. Neither study specifically examined dopamine neuronal systems, mesencephalon, or striatum.

As extensively reviewed by Feldman,[32] acute exposure to TCE in people has been reported to cause dizziness, headache, nausea, vomiting, alcohol intolerance, loss of consciousness, cranial nerve V neuropathy, multiple cranial neuropathies, and peripheral neuropathy. Chronic exposure can cause dizziness, fatigue, headache, irritability, sleep disturbance, impaired memory/concentration, paresthesias, alcohol intolerance, peripheral neuropathy, impaired attention and executive functioning, short-term memory problems, visuospatial disability, discoordination, and tremor.

HUMAN CASES AND EPIDEMIOLOGIC STUDIES

An occupational study of TCE vapor emissions in a pump room was reported by Vandervort and Polnkoff in 1973.[50] Workers were exposed for an average of 8 years. Common complaints included eye irritation, dizziness, drowsiness, weakness, cough, and palpitations. Multiple case reports reveal a wide range of clinical manifestations due to exposure to TCE.[32] Chronic exposure is considered to be a significant risk factor for cancer; the World Health Organization International Agency for Research on Cancer (IARC) classifies TCE as a probable (group 2A) human carcinogen.[51,52]

In 1999, Guehl reported a case of a 47-year-old woman who was professionally exposed to TCE for several months in an uncontrolled and unprotected environment.[53] She was a house cleaner and worked with TCE in poorly ventilated rooms. Later, she worked in the plastics industry where she was exposed to multiple solvents including TCE. She was diagnosed with parkinsonism in 1987, after 7 years of exposure.

Gash and colleagues[54] in 2008 reported a group of industrial workers who were variously exposed to TCE for 8 to 33 years and subsequently diagnosed with iPD or parkinsonian features. A questionnaire was mailed to 134 former workers, of whom 65 responded. Twenty-one self-reported at least 3 Parkinson signs/symptoms (slowness of voluntary movement, stooped posture, trouble with balance, slow walk or dragging feet, rigidity or stiffness, tremor, decreased facial expression); 23 respondents reported 1 to 2 signs/symptoms, and 21 reported no signs/symptoms. Fourteen of the 21 workers reporting at least 3 signs/symptoms and 13 coworkers without self-reported signs agreed to further participation in the study. The most common routes of exposure were inhalation and dermal. At the time of the study 3 workers with chronic dermal and inhalation exposure to TCE had been diagnosed with iPD; many coworkers displayed features of parkinsonism. This observation suggested a relationship between the TCE exposure and development of iPD, parkinsonian features, and other movement disorders including tics and tremors.

Goldman studied TCE exposure in a population of twin pairs discordant for iPD. An industrial hygienist reviewed histories and solvent exposures from the age 10 years until the diagnosis of iPD in the affected twin. It was concluded from this study that risk of iPD was increased more than fivefold in twins who had been occupationally exposed to TCE. This population-based epidemiologic study further supported the role of TCE exposure in the development of iPD.[55]

Animal Studies

After a sentinel case of iPD in a worker exposed to TCE (see section on human cases and epidemiology studies), Guehl and colleagues[53] studied TCE exposure in mice and dopaminergic neurotoxicity. After exposing mice to either TCE or saline, via intraperitoneal injection for 4 weeks, they examined the midbrains of these mice. There was a significant decrease in the number of tyrosine hydroxylase (TH) immunoreactive neurons in TCE-treated mice compared with saline-treated mice. Following up on their human epidemiologic studies, Gash and colleagues exposed 5-month-old male Fisher 344 rats to TCE.[54,56] Animals were orally administered doses of 200, 500 or 1000 mg/kg TCE in 0.6 mL olive oil, or they received vehicle by oral gavage once a day, 5 days per week for 6 weeks. TCE serum concentration at the highest doses was 55 to 60 µg/mL, compared with estimated TCE blood levels of dry cleaning workers that may range up to 1.7 µg/mL. The goal was to replicate in days or weeks what may require years of exposure in people. TH immunochemistry was performed in the substantia nigra, and the total numbers of TH-positive cells were counted. There was a dose-dependent loss of dopaminergic neurons in substantia nigra, from 20.1% at the lowest to 40.6% loss at the highest TCE concentration exposure. No significant obvious neuronal loss was noted in locus coeruleus and dorsal motor nucleus of vagus nerve, both of which undergo neurodegeneration in iPD. No damage to the Purkinje cells in cerebellum was noted. Hence TCE exposure caused selective loss of neurons in the nigrostriatal system.[56]

Levels of monoamines and their metabolites were also measured in the nigrostriatal system. It was demonstrated that striatal levels of the dopamine metabolites 3,4-dihydroxyphenylacetic acid (DOPAC) and homovanillic acid (HVA) were significantly reduced in TCE-treated rats, whereas dopamine levels were not altered.[56] Similar findings were observed in mice treated for 3 weeks with the herbicide paraquat; the authors speculated this was due to compensatory mechanisms in striatum, where they demonstrated enhanced TH activity.[57] Serotonin and its metabolites were not affected in the sampling sites that included striatum and substantia nigra. Behavioral and locomotor studies, including rotarod performance and spontaneous locomotor activity, demonstrated parkinsonian-like motor deficits in TCE-treated animals.[56]

To determine if TCE-induced neurodegeneration was associated with mitochondrial dysfunction, mitochondrial enzyme activity was measured. In treated animals, there was selective inhibition of mitochondrial complex 1 enzyme activity that led to depletion of adenosine triphosphate (ATP). Levels of caspase 3 were significantly higher in TCE-exposed rats and this, together with ATP depletion, was considered to be responsible for apoptosis. Moreover, tyrosine nitration and activated microglial cells were also observed in neurons in substantia nigra. The authors concluded mitochondrial complex 1 enzyme dysfunction, increased levels of apoptotic enzymes, oxidative and nitrative stress, and inflammation were all implicated in the pathogenic mechanism of TCE-induced parkinsonism. Of note, immunostaining was also performed to determine the accumulation of alpha-synuclein in neurons. Increased accumulations of intracellular alpha-synuclein were noted in dorsal motor nucleus of vagus nerve and in the substantia nigra pars compacta in the TCE-exposed group.[56] All the potential pathogenetic mechanisms activated by exposure to TCE most likely act in concert to create a vicious downward spiral that ultimately leads to neurodegeneration, particularly but probably not exclusively in substantia nigra.

SUMMARY

A combination of potential risk (eg, exposure to pesticides, herbicides, heavy metals) and protective (eg, use of nicotine, caffeine) factors has been associated with the development of iPD, as has underlying genetic susceptibility.[58] Among these, TCE exposure appears to be a risk factor based on recent observations associating chronic TCE exposure and development of iPD or parkinsonian features.[54,55] Clearly, TCE exposure alone is insufficient, as some individuals appear to have developed frank iPD while others with similar exposure have been asymptomatic or have presented with mild motor abnormalities that, although insufficient to make the diagnosis of iPD, included tremors and rigidity.[54] Animal models of TCE exposure that produce an iPD phenotype strengthen this potential link.[56] TCE has been shown to induce nigrostriatal degeneration by mitochondrial dysfunction, oxidative/nitrative stress, and neuroinflammation. Whether this is due to a direct effect of TCE or mediated through a metabolite, particularly TaClo, is not known. Regardless, a credible hypothesis develops that chronic exposure to TCE can lead to the degeneration of the nigrostriatal dopaminergic system and clinical parkinsonism. Therefore, safety measures for TCE should be observed in work places and enforced for the general environment.

REFERENCES

1. Vance JM, Ali S, Bradley WG, et al. Gene–environment interactions in Parkinson's disease and other forms of parkinsonism. Neurotoxicology 2010;31(5):598–602.
2. Nagatsu T, Sawada M. Cellular and molecular mechanisms of Parkinson's disease: neurotoxins, causative genes, and inflammatory cytokines. Cell Mol Neurobiol 2006;26:781–802.
3. Fall PA, Fredrikson M, Axelson O, et al. Nutritional and occupational factors influencing the risk of Parkinson's disease: a case–control study in southeastern Sweden. Mov Disord 1999;14(1):28–37.
4. Gorell JM, Johnson CC, Rybicki BA, et al. Occupational exposures to metals as risk factors for Parkinson's disease. Neurology 1997;48(3):650–8.
5. Zorzon M, Capus L, Pellegrino A, et al. Familial and environmental risk factors in Parkinson's disease: a case–control study in northeast Italy. Acta Neurol Scand 2002;105(2):77–82.
6. Langston JW. The impact of MPTP on Parkinson's disease research: past, present, and future. In: Factor SA, Weiner WJ, editors. Parkinson's disease: diagnosis and clinical management. 2nd edition. New York: Demos; 2008. p. 407–36.
7. Priyadarshi A, Khuder SA, Schaub EA, et al. A meta-analysis of Parkinson's disease and exposure to pesticides. Neurotoxicology 2000;21(4):435–40.
8. Tanner CM. Occupational and environmental causes of parkinsonism. In: Shusterman D, Blanc P, editors. Occupational medicine: state of the art reviews. Philadelphia: Hanley & Belfus; 1992. p. 503–13.
9. Gorell JM, Johnson CC, Rybicki BA, et al. The risk of Parkinson's disease with exposure to pesticides, farming, well water, and rural living. Neurology 1998;50(5):1346–50.
10. Lin MT, Beal MF. Mitochondrial dysfunction and oxidative stress in neurodegenerative diseases. Nature 2006;443(7113):787–95.
11. Li W, Lesuisse C, Xu Y, et al. Stabilization of alpha-synuclein protein with aging and familial Parkinson's disease-linked A53T mutation. J Neurosci 2004;24(33): 7400–9.
12. Manning-Bog AB, McCormack AL, Li J, et al. The herbicide paraquat causes up-regulation and aggregation of alpha-synuclein in mice: paraquat and alpha-synuclein. J Biol Chem 2002;277(3):1641–4.
13. Purisai MG, McCormack AL, Langston WJ, et al. Alpha-synuclein expression in the substantia nigra of MPTP-lesioned nonhuman primates. Neurobiol Dis 2005; 20(3):898–906.

14. Zhu J, Chu CT. Mitochondrial dysfunction in Parkinson's disease. J Alzheimers Dis 2010;20(Suppl 2):S325–34.
15. Langston JW, Ballard P, Tetrud JW, et al. Chronic parkinsonism in humans due to a product of meperidine-analog synthesis. Science 1983;219(4587):979–80.
16. Betarbet R, Sherer TB, MacKenzie G, et al. Chronic systemic pesticide exposure reproduces features of Parkinson's disease. Nat Neurosci 2000;3(12): 1301–6.
17. Perier C, Bove J, Vila M, et al. The rotenone model of Parkinson's disease. Trends Neurosci 2003;26(7):345–6.
18. Haas RH, Nasirian F, Nakano K, et al. Low platelet mitochondrial complex I and complex II/III activity in early untreated Parkinson's disease. Ann Neurol 1995; 37(6):714–22.
19. Parker WD Jr, Boyson SJ, Parks JK. Abnormalities of the electron transport chain in idiopathic Parkinson's disease. Ann Neurol 1989;26(6):719–23.
20. Parker WD Jr, Parks JK, Swerdlow RH. Complex I deficiency in Parkinson's disease frontal cortex. Brain Res 2008;1189:215–8.
21. Mizukawa K, Sora YH, Ogawa N. Ultrastructural changes of the substantia nigra, ventral tegmental area and striatum in 1-methyl-4-phenyl-1,2,3,6-tetrahydropyridine (MPTP)-treated mice. Res Commun Chem Pathol Pharmacol 1990;67(3): 307–20.
22. Rapisardi SC, Warrington VO, Wilson JS. Effects of MPTP on the fine structure of neurons in substantia nigra of dogs. Brain Res 1990;512(1):147–54.
23. Tanaka J, Nakamura H, Honda S, et al. Neuropathological study on 1-methyl-4-phenyl-1,2,3,6-tetrahydropyridine of the crab-eating monkey. Acta Neuropathol 1988;75(4):370–6.
24. Trimmer PA, Swerdlow RH, Parks JK, et al. Abnormal mitochondrial morphology in sporadic Parkinson's and Alzheimer's disease cybrid cell lines. Exp Neurol 2000;162(1):37–50.
25. Song DD, Shults CW, Sisk A, et al. Enhanced substantia nigra mitochondrial pathology in human alpha-synuclein transgenic mice after treatment with MPTP. Exp Neurol 2004;186(2):158–72.
26. Zhu JH, Horbinski C, Guo F, et al. Regulation of autophagy by extracellular signal-regulated protein kinases during 1-methyl-4-phenylpyridinium-induced cell death. Am J Pathol 2007;170(1):75–86.
27. McCrank E, Rabheru K. Four cases of progressive supranuclear palsy in patients exposed to organic solvents. Can J Psychiatry 1989;34(9):934–6.
28. Uitti RJ, Snow BJ, Shinotoh H, et al. Parkinsonism induced by solvent abuse. Ann Neurol 1994;35(5):616–9.
29. Doherty RE. A history of the production and use of carbon tetrachloride, tetrachloroethylene, trichloroethylene, and 1,1,1-trichloroethane in the United States: part 2-trichloroethylene and 1,1,1-trichloroethane. J Environmental Forensics 2000;1(2): 83–93.
30. Kroschwitz J, Howe-Grant M. Kirk-Othmer Encyclopedia of Chemical Technology. New York: Wiley & Sons; 1991.
31. Williams-Johnson M, Eisenmann CJ, Donkin SG, et al. Toxicological profile for trichloroethylene. Atlanta (GA): Agency for Toxic Substances and Disease Registry; 1997.
32. Feldman RG. Occupational & environmental neurotoxicology. Philadelphia: Lippincott-Raven; 1999.
33. Trichloroethylene CoHHRo. Assessing the human health risks of trichloroethylene: key scientific issues. Washington, DC: The National Academies Press; 2006.

34. Bringmann G, Hille A. Endogenous alkaloids in man, VII: 1-trichloromethyl-1,2,3,4-tetrahydro-beta-carboline–a potential chloral-derived indol alkaloid in man. Arch Pharm (Weinheim) 1990;323(9):567–9.

35. Bringmann G, God R, Feineis D, et al. TaClo as a neurotoxic lead: improved synthesis, stereochemical analysis, and inhibition of the mitochondrial respiratory chain. J Neural Transm Suppl 1995;46:245–54.

36. Bringmann G, God R, Feineis D, et al. The TaClo concept: 1-trichloromethyl-1,2,3,4-tetrahydro-beta-carboline (TaClo), a new toxin for dopaminergic neurons. J Neural Transm Suppl 1995;46:235–44.

37. Kochen W, Kohlmuller D, De Biasi P, et al. The endogeneous formation of highly chlorinated tetrahydro-beta-carbolines as a possible causative mechanism in idiopathic Parkinson's disease. Adv Exp Med Biol 2003;527:253–63.

38. Rausch WD, Abdel-mohsen M, Koutsilieri E, et al. Studies of the potentially endogenous toxin TaClo (1-trichloromethyl-1,2,3,4-tetrahydro-beta-carboline) in neuronal and glial cell cultures. J Neural Transm Suppl 1995;46:255–63.

39. Janetzky B, Gille D, Abdel-Mohsen M, et al. Effect of highly halogenated h-carbolines on dopaminergic cells in culture and on mitochondrial respiration. Drug Dev Res 1999;46:51–6.

40. Bringmann G, Feineis D, God R, et al. Neurotoxic effects on the dopaminergic system induced by TaClo (1-trichloromethyl-1,2,3,4-tetrahydro-β-carboline), a potential mammalian alkaloid: in vivo and in vitro studies. Biog Amines 1996;12:83–102.

41. Grote C, Clement HW, Wesemann W, et al. Biochemical lesions of the nigrostriatal system by TaClo (1-trichloromethyl-1,2,3,4-tetrahydro-beta-carboline) and derivatives. J Neural Transm Suppl 1995;46:275–81.

42. Riederer P, Foley P, Bringmann G, et al. Biochemical and pharmacological characterization of 1-trichloromethyl-1,2,3,4-tetrahydro-beta-carboline: a biologically relevant neurotoxin? Eur J Pharmacol 2002;442:1–16.

43. Bringmann G, Feineis D, Bruckner R, et al. Synthesis of radiolabelled 1-trichloromethyl-1,2,3,4-tetrahydro-beta-carboline (TaClo), a neurotoxic chloral-derived mammalian alkaloid, and its biodistribution in rats. Eur J Pharm Sci Aug 2006;28(5):412–22.

44. Drucker G, Raikoff K, Neafsey EJ, et al. Dopamine uptake inhibitory capacities of beta-carboline and 3,4-dihydro-beta-carboline analogs of N-methyl-4-phenyl-1,2,3,6-tetrahydropyridine (MPTP) oxidation products. Brain Res 1990;509(1):125–33.

45. McNaught KS, Thull U, Carrupt PA, et al. Inhibition of [3H]dopamine uptake into striatal synaptosomes by isoquinoline derivatives structurally related to 1-methyl-4-phenyl-1,2,3,6-tetrahydropyridine. Biochem Pharmacol 1996;52(1):29–34.

46. Akundi RS, Macho A, Munoz E, et al. 1-trichloromethyl-1,2,3,4-tetrahydro-beta-carboline-induced apoptosis in the human neuroblastoma cell line SK-N-SH. J Neurochem 2004;91(2):263–73.

47. Janetzky B, God R, Bringmann G, et al. 1-Trichloromethyl-1,2,3,4-tetrahydro-beta-carboline, a new inhibitor of complex I. J Neural Transm Suppl 1995;46:265–73.

48. Haglid KG, Briving C, Hansson HA, et al. Trichloroethylene: long-lasting changes in the brain after rehabilitation. Neurotoxicology 1981;2(4):659–73.

49. Briving C, Jacobson I, Hamberger A, et al. Chronic effects of perchloroethylene and trichloroethylene on the gerbil brain amino acids and glutathione. Neurotoxicology 1986;7(1):101–8.

50. Vandervort R, Polnkoff P. Dunham-Bush, Inc, West Hartford, CN (Health hazard evaluation/toxicity determination report 72-84-31; US NTIS PB-229-627). Cincinnati (OH): National Institute for Occupational Safety and Health; 1973.
51. Trichloroethylene. IARC monographs on the evaluation of the carcinogenic risk of chemicals to humans. vol. 20. Lyon (France): International Agency for Research on Cancer; 1979. p. 545–72.
52. Dry cleaning, some chlorinated solvents and other industrial chemicals. IARC monographs on the evaluation of carcinogenic risk of chemicals to humans, vol. 63. Lyon (France): International Agency for Research on Cancer; 1995. p. 75–158.
53. Guehl D, Bezard E, Dovero S, et al. Trichloroethylene and parkinsonism: a human and experimental observation. Eur J Neurol 1999;6(5):609–11.
54. Gash DM, Rutland K, Hudson NL, et al. Trichloroethylene: parkinsonism and complex 1 mitochondrial neurotoxicity. Ann Neurol 2008;63(2):184–92.
55. Goldman SM. Trichloroethylene and Parkinson's disease: dissolving the puzzle. Expert Rev Neurother 2010;10(6):835–7.
56. Liu M, Choi DY, Hunter RL, et al. Trichloroethylene induces dopaminergic neurodegeneration in Fisher 344 rats. J Neurochem 2010;112(3):773–83.
57. McCormack AL, Thiruchelvam M, Manning-Bog AB, et al. Environmental risk factors and Parkinson's disease: selective degeneration of nigral dopaminergic neurons caused by the herbicide paraquat. Neurobiol Dis 2002;10(2):119–27.
58. Chade AR, Kasten M, Tanner CM. Nongenetic causes of Parkinson's disease. J Neural Transm Suppl 2006;(70):147–51.

Neurotoxic Pesticides and Neurologic Effects

David A. Jett, PhD

KEYWORDS

• Pesticides • Neurologic effects • Neurologic diseases

ANTICHOLINESTERASE INSECTICIDES

Case Study 1

A 75-year-old woman ingested a large quantity of the pesticide Dy-Syston, which contains the organophosphate disulfoton.[1] The woman began to experience diarrhea and vomiting, and was admitted to the hospital, where gastric lavage was immediately performed. At this time, only muscle fasciculations were apparent, but 90 minutes after admission, confusion, severe miosis, and cardiac arrhythmia were observed. Erythrocyte cholinesterase was depressed at 3524 IU/L (normal 10,000–14,000 IU/L), as was plasma cholinesterase at 181 IU/L. Atropine sulfate and pralidoxime (2-PAM) were infused intravenously, atropine at 1 mg every 30 minutes, and 2-PAM at 0.5 g/h.

Phosphorodithioate sulfone, a more toxic metabolite of disulfoton, was present in plasma but decreased 20 hours after admission. Sulfone concentrations in plasma rebounded on day 3, causing a concomitant decrease in erythrocyte cholinesterase. Sulfone concentrations then dropped precipitously, and the plasma cholinesterase concentration increased in the next 2 weeks with continued gastric lavage and atropine/2-PAM infusion. Symptoms of cholinergic intoxication also subsided, even in the presence of continued depression of erythrocyte cholinesterase. The patient showed complete recovery by day 28.

Case Study 2

A 22-year-old pregnant woman (29th week) presented having had several generalized tonic-clonic seizures.[2] An initial diagnosis of eclampsia was made and treatment with intravenous MgSO$_4$ was initiated. The signs of anticholinesterase toxicity included vomiting, diarrhea, hypersecretions within the airways, pinpoint pupils, and muscle weakness and fasciculations. After intravenous doses of atropine, the patient responded and survived. The infant was born prematurely and died 2 days after birth without showing any signs of cholinergic crises or organophosphate intoxication.

A version of this article originally appeared in *Dobbs MR, editor. Clinical Neurotoxicology. Philadelphia: Elsevier; 2009.*

The information in this article is provided for educational purposes only and does not necessarily represent endorsement by, or an official position of, the National Institute of Neurologic Disorders and Stroke or any other Federal agency.

Office of Translational Research, National Institute of Neurological Disorders and Stroke, National Institutes of Health, 6001 Executive Boulevard, NSC, Room 2177, MSC 9527, Bethesda, MD 20892-9527, USA

E-mail address: jettd@ninds.nih.gov

Anticholinesterase pesticides inhibit the hydrolytic enzyme acetylcholinesterase (AChE) (BC 3.1.1.7). The most common of these are esters of phosphoric or phosphorothioic acid. Commonly referred to as the organophosphates (OPs), this group is a large, chemically diverse class that includes more than 200 compounds containing one of a dozen or more different organophosphorus esters (**Fig. 1**). Most are insecticides, but there are OP, carbamate herbicides, and fungicides that are nontoxic to humans. Related to the OP insecticides are the organophosphorus nerve gases developed for chemical warfare during World War II, which include the highly toxic VX and sarin (see **Fig. 1**). Another important class of pesticides is the carbamates, which are carbamic acid esters with an anticholinesterase mode of action that is similar to that of the OPs. These compounds are used as insecticides, fungicides, and herbicides. They inhibit cholinesterases by way of their carbamoyl and thiocarbamoyl structure.

OP insecticides are effective because of their ability to phosphorylate and deactivate AChE. This enzyme is also carbamylated by carbamate pesticides that produce similar effects. In mammalian systems, the acute toxicity of OP and carbamate insecticides is derived from this anticholinesterase activity and subsequent parasympathomimetic effects. AChE is an essential hydrolytic enzyme found in the central nervous system and the autonomic systems of the peripheral nervous system, and at all neuromuscular junctions. OPs and other anticholinesterases acylate the enzyme at the esteratic site, as does its substrate, the neurotransmitter acetylcholine (ACh). A major difference between the OPs and carbamates is the rate of dephosphorylation or decarbamoylation of the inhibited enzyme. The carbamates are largely reversible because of a fast rate of deacylation, whereas the rate is so slow with OPs that they are considered irreversible, and consequently they require more extensive medical intervention.

Some OPs and carbamates also interact with another enzyme, termed neuropathy target esterase (NTE). This is believed to be the initiating event for the development of

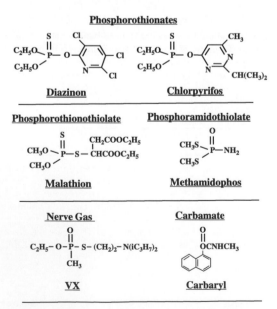

Fig. 1. Typical organophosphate and carbamate insecticides and nerve gases.

a delayed polyneuropathy called organophosphate-induced delayed neuropathy (OPIDN).[3] The acute and chronic toxicity of OPs has been studied extensively in laboratory animal models and in occupationally exposed humans; this has been reviewed elsewhere.[4] Some OPs can be transferred to the fetus via the placenta and are teratogenic, causing various abnormalities such as growth retardation, micromelia, and axial skeletal problems, and this may have serious implications for the health of children exposed to low to moderate levels.[4,5] These studies and evidence of extensive human exposures in some areas have led to concern that public health may be affected adversely by their extensive commercial and residential use. OPs are also believed to act as immunosuppressants, primarily through alteration of macrophage function.[4] Some of the toxicity may be modified with continuous exposure. Tolerance to OPs develops as a result of compensatory responses involving the downregulation of cholinergic receptors and responses.

Most cases of acute poisoning from anticholinesterase pesticides are from suicide attempts. Signs of acute intoxication by these compounds depend on the severity of exposure, and they reflect their anticholinesterase activity at muscarinic and nicotinic cholinergic synapses. The muscarinic effects are primarily parasympathomimetic and are manifested in the lung, gastrointestinal system, sweat glands, salivary glands, lacrimal glands, cardiovascular system, pupils, and bladder. With some OPs, pancreatitis may occur and lead to fatality, often without any pain or other indications. Other effects on the sympathetic nervous system and somatic motor nerves are a result of overstimulation of nicotinic cholinergic receptors. A mnemonic used in the diagnosis of anticholinesterases that incorporates the hallmark signs of intoxication is DUMBELS, for diarrhea, urination, miosis, bronchospasm, emesis, lacrimation, salivation (**Fig. 2**). Other muscarinic effects include tightness in the chest, wheezing, rhinitis, dyspnea, increased bronchial secretions, pulmonary edema, cyanosis, nausea, tenesmus, sweating, and blurred vision. Other nicotinic effects are muscular twitching and fasciculations, weakness, cramps, and pallor.

Chronic neurologic sequelae may result from acute OP poisoning, possibly as a result of the initiation of neurodegenerative processes by excitotoxic responses. There is some evidence that Gulf War veterans and victims of the terrorist attacks in Japan may have suffered long-term effects from exposures to nerve agents and pesticides.[6,7] Chronic exposures may result in 2 distinct syndromes: OPIDN, and one that results in symptoms that are intermediate between OPIDN and acute effects. The intermediate syndrome appears between the appearance of signs of acute poisoning and the onset of delayed polyneuropathies associated with OPIDN. It is characterized by respiratory paresis and motor cranial nerve weakness, and can lead to death from respiratory failure. OPIDN is related not to inhibition of AChE, but

Diarrhea

Urination

Miosis

Bronchospasm

Emesis

Lacrimation

Salivation

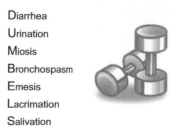

Fig. 2. Signs and symptoms of organophosphate toxicity.

to inhibition of NTE. Consequently, respiratory muscles are spared, but flaccid weakness and atrophy of distal limbs, spasticity, and ataxia are diagnostic of a delayed sensorimotor polyneuropathy.[8] Many of the neuropsychological effects of low-level exposure seem to involve the cognitive processes that underlie learning and memory. Some people exposed to these compounds may experience memory loss even in the absence of overt toxicity or significant cholinesterase inhibition.

The diagnosis of acute poisoning from anticholinesterases is based on the presence of the compounds or metabolites in available biologic samples, inhibition of AChE, cholinergic signs of intoxication, and response to treatment with atropine and 2-PAM. Diazepam is also used for reducing anxiety in mild poisoning cases, and it can control muscle fasiculations and convulsions in more severe cases. The diagnosis of chronic poisoning from laboratory data is more difficult because of the uncoupling of chronic toxicity to AChE inhibition. AChE inhibition is present in the intermediate syndrome of OP poisoning, but not with OPIDN. Laboratory analysis of AChE activity can be determined in red blood cells and butyrylcholinesterase can be determined in plasma, but it does not always correlate well with AChE.

ORGANOCHLORINE INSECTICIDES

> *Case Study 3*
>
> A 13-month-old boy was found with an open bottle of Kwell lotion (1% lindane), with some of the contents in his mouth and on his clothes.[9] The child vomited twice and had a generalized tonic-clonic seizure before being transported to the hospital. After having another seizure in the hospital, he was given phenobarbital, underwent gastric lavage, and was given activated charcoal. His respiratory effort diminished, and he was intubated. Urinalysis results were normal, and his blood lindane concentrations were 0.32 µg/mL 4 hours after ingestion, and 0.02 µg/mL 20 hours after ingestion. The child was extubated 8 hours later, and his condition improved over the next 2 days, at which time he was discharged.

The organochlorine (OC) insecticides (also called chlorinated hydrocarbons) are neurotoxic and have several other harmful effects related to their estrogenic properties. Most were banned from use in the United States in the 1970s. This was primarily due to evidence that these compounds have carcinogenic properties, and their ability to accumulate and cause harmful effects in wildlife. Insect resistance to many of the compounds played a much less publicized role in the decline in use of OC insecticides. Currently there is debate on the global cost of tougher regulations on these compounds relative to their beneficial role in controlling insect-borne diseases such as malaria. DDT (dichlorodiphenyltrichloroethane) is a major part of programs to eradicate mosquito larvae, and is still used as a human delousing agent and as an inexpensive agricultural insecticide in some parts of the world. Several methods of classification may be used to describe the OC insecticides, and a more extensive review of their toxicology is presented elsewhere.[10] One structural classification includes the dichlorodiphenylethanes, DDT, the cyclodienes (eg, dieldrin), and the cyclohexanes (eg, lindane) (**Fig. 3**). The cyclodienes are extremely toxic as a group, and they have diverse chemical structure and toxicity. The cyclohexanes are among the oldest synthetic insecticides, and many are isomers of hexachlorocyclohexane. Lindane is the y-isomer (see **Fig. 3**).

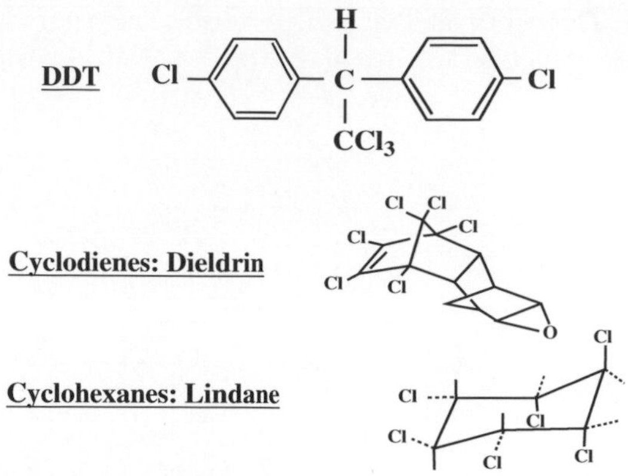

DDT

Cyclodienes: Dieldrin

Cyclohexanes: Lindane

Fig. 3. Typical organochlorine insecticides.

The OCs are absorbed readily by the body and stored for extended periods in adipose tissues. The cyclodienes and cyclohexanes have resulted in several fatalities because they are readily absorbed through the skin. Although banned by the Environmental Protection Agency (EPA) in 2006 for agricultural use, lindane is used topically to treat scabies and in shampoo to combat lice in cases where alternative treatments are either not well tolerated or ineffective. Lindane exposure has resulted in serious illness and deaths when used improperly (Case Study 3). The primary urinary metabolite of DDT in humans is dideoxyadenosine, or DDA [bis(p-chlorophenyl)acetic acid]. One of the more important metabolites is dichlorodiphenyldichloroethylene, or DDE [1,1-dichloro-2,2-bis(p-chlorophenyl)ethylene] because it may be stored in adipose tissues for decades. The putative link between this compound and breast cancer in humans has not been well supported, however, the role of DDE in human disease has not been dismissed and is still under investigation.[11] The metabolism of OCs is slow compared with other pesticides, due in part to the complex ring structure and extent of chlorination. The slow metabolism, high lipid solubility, and persistence in adipose tissue are why the OCs are still of concern to health care professionals.

The OC insecticides are acutely neurotoxic. The mechanism of action is best understood where they interfere with neurotransmission at the level of the nerve synapse. DDT interferes with the function of sodium channels by prolonging the falling phase of the action potential, leading to repetitive firing of the nerve impulse.[12] This, along with an interaction with axonal ATPases and calmodulin, causes hyperexcitability. The mechanism of toxicity for the cyclodienes and cyclohexanes is by interference with γ-aminobutyric acid (GABA) neurotransmission through inhibition of GABA receptors and blockage of voltage-gated chloride channels. The OC insecticides can be divided into 2 groups based on their mode of action: tremorogenic compounds that act on sodium channels (eg, DDT and related compounds) and convulsant compounds that act on GABA receptors (cyclodienes, lindane).

The signs and symptoms of poisoning from OC insecticides are outlined in **Box 1**. The signs from acute exposure are due to the alteration of ion channels causing neuronal hyperexcitability. Hallmark signs and symptoms of OC exposure differ somewhat between the tremorogenic DDT and the convulsant lindane and cyclodiene class, but there is some significant overlap (see **Box 1**). Other signs of DDT exposure include numbness and, in rare cases, convulsions. Acute effects in addition to those listed in **Box 1** include hearing whistling noises, seeing colored lights, visual

---

Box 1
Signs and symptoms of organochlorine insecticide poisoning

Acute Effects

- Tremor
- Paresthesia
- Ataxia
- Dizziness
- Nausea
- Convulsions
- Hyperexcitability
- Hyperflexia
- Myclonic jerking
- General malaise

Chronic Effects

- Weight loss
- Anemia
- Tremors
- Weakness
- Electroencephalogram changes
- Hyperexcitability
- Nervousness
- Psychological
- Arthralgia
- Low spermatogenesis
- Visual difficulty
- Memory loss
- Skin rash

---

impairment, giddiness, headache preceding mixed-type seizures, confusion, and speech difficulties. The cyclodienes, including dieldrin, chlordane, and the once widely used toxaphene, may also cause hypothermia, anorexia, epigastric pain, and vomiting. Seizures from acute OC exposure may be delayed and may not occur for as long as 6 to 8 months after exposure.

Chronic exposure to OCs is of particular importance because of their long half-lives in human adipose tissues. In addition to the tremors, weight loss, and anemia caused by prolonged exposure to DDT (see **Box 1**), dicofol (a DDT analogue), may cause headache, blurred vision, numbness, and other psychological changes and cognitive deficits.[8] Other chronic signs of lindane and cyclodiene exposure are headache, dizziness, myoclonic jerking, chest pain, ataxia, loss of coordination, and slurred speech. Chlordecone (Kepone) was studied extensively after industrial workers in Hopewell, VA, USA were exposed through poor industrial hygiene.[13]

PYRETHROID INSECTICIDES

Case Study 4

A 44-year-old woman who had been using cans of pyrethroid insecticides almost every day for 3 years in an unventilated room experienced tongue numbness, nausea, and rhinitis while using the insecticides.[14] After 2 years, she had difficulty lifting heavy objects with her left arm, and her symptoms steadily worsened over the next 8 months. Three months before admission to the hospital, she developed slurred speech, gait disturbance, and generalized muscle weakness. On admission, neurologic examination revealed dysarthria, nasal voice, and dysphagia with fasciculations and moderate muscle weakness. Sensory and autonomic systems were all normal. Nerve conduction studies showed decreased compound muscle action potentials amplitudes and motor-evoked potentials revealed prolonged central conduction time. Two months after cessation of pesticide use, her motor weakness partially ameliorated and fasciculation in all 4 limbs ceased. A subclinical hypothyroidism seen on admission had also improved, and 7 months after cessation of pesticide use, no exacerbation was apparent.

Like many insecticides, the pyrethroids target the nervous systems of insects so that rapid incapacitating and killing function is maximized. The botanic pyrethroid insecticides are synthetic analogues of pyrethrins extracted from pyrethrum flowers of the genus *Chrysanthemum*. The pyrethrins have been used as insecticides for more than a century, but large-scale agricultural and home use has been facilitated by efforts over the past few decades to synthesize less expensive analogues with better stability in the environment. The synthetic pyrethroids have remarkable knock-down insecticidal properties and have retained some, but not all, of the chemical properties that made the pyrethrins virtually nontoxic to mammals. The general structure of pyrethroids resembles that of pyrethrins, which are composed of esters of 2 carboxylic acids, chrysanthemic acid and pyrethric acid (**Fig. 4**).

The pyrethroids are among the least toxic pesticides to mammals. Systemic toxicity of these compounds is usually associated with oral or inhalation exposures. Absorption through the skin is minimal. Many of the reported occupational and home poisonings are of the result of allergic reactions to dermal exposures accompanied by rashes and paresthesia. Like the OP and the OC pesticides, the pyrethroids are nerve poisons. The pyrethroids and DDT have remarkably similar effects on voltage-gated sodium channels. The action of pyrethroids on sodium channels causes repetitive neuronal discharge and the neuronal hyperexcitability characteristic of nerve excitants.

Two distinct classes of pyrethroid insecticides have been identified based on specific sets of symptoms they produce in laboratory rats. The T syndrome, or Type I poisoning, is characterized primarily by tremor, and results from exposure to

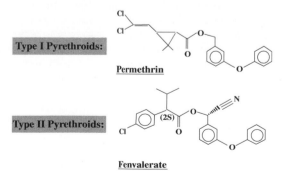

Type I Pyrethroids:

Permethrin

Type II Pyrethroids:

Fenvalerate

Fig. 4. Typical pyrethroid insecticides.

compounds without the α-cyano substituent. Acute symptoms are virtually indistinguishable from DDT intoxication. Other related symptoms in laboratory animals observed with Type I pyrethroids are aggression, restlessness, muscle twitches, hyperexcitability, incoordination, and prostration. The Type II pyrethroids possess the α-cyano group and produce the CS syndrome characterized by choreoathetosis (C) and salivation (S). The CS syndrome may also produce an increase in coarse whole-body tremors, but they progress to sinuous writhing and seizures. A reaction to dermal exposure to pyrethroids may result in cutaneous paresthesia, which has been observed with pyrethrins and with Type I and II pyrethroids. To date, there has been no conclusive evidence to suggest that environmental exposures to pyrethroids produce chronic toxicity. However, the number of pyrethrin and pyrethroid-related poisoning incidents in children has been increasing,[15] and with their widespread use, children in daycare centers have been reported to be exposed to several pyrethroid pesticides.[16]

PESTICIDE EXPOSURES AND NEUROLOGIC DISEASE

Historically, most emphasis on the neurotoxic effects of pesticides has been focused on neurologic symptoms following high-level acute exposures. However, recent interest has focused on the possibility that long-term low-level exposures to pesticides may be involved in the development of persistent neurologic deficits and several neurologic diseases including Parkinson disease (PD), Alzheimer disease (AD), and amyotrophic lateral sclerosis (ALS).[17] Several studies have identified pesticide exposure as a risk factor for PD.[18] The pesticide paraquat has been studied extensively as a model for PD[19,20]; other pesticides such as maneb and rotenone have also been linked to the development of PD.

Other studies have demonstrated that drinking well-water and living in a rural setting, both of which may increase exposure to agricultural pesticides, increase the risk of developing PD. Flemming and colleagues[21] demonstrated that the presence of the organochlorine dieldrin in postmortem brain tissue was significantly associated with the diagnosis of PD. This observation has recently been confirmed by Corrigan and colleagues,[22] who observed elevated levels of dieldrin and lindane in postmortem samples of substantia nigra taken from patients with PD. However, both of these studies suffered from small sample sizes (>20). A larger study found dieldrin exposure was a risk factor for PD in humans more so than other pesticides.[23] A large multicenter clinical study found that exposure to any one of several pesticides with mechanisms linked to experimental PD was a risk factor.[24] In all likelihood, PD is a multifactorial disease and both environmental and genetic factors are important.[25,26] The environmental factors are not necessarily limited to pesticides, and include other dopaminergic toxins such as manganese.[27]

There are much less data with regard to pesticide exposure as a potential risk factor for AD. Santibanez and colleagues[28] reviewed several of the epidemiologic studies that have looked at environmental risk factors for AD and concluded that of the 6 studies that explored the possible relationship between pesticide exposure and AD, there was sufficient evidence from prospective design studies to conclude there was a significant relationship between pesticide exposure and risk of AD. For example, Baldi and colleagues[29] found an adjusted risk ratio of 2.39 for AD in men occupationally exposed to pesticides. However, these studies suffered from lack of identification of specific pesticides as many of the epidemiologic studies do with regard to neurodegenerative disease. In a study of more than 3000 enrollees, pesticide exposure was associated with dementia and AD later in life.[30]

With regard to ALS, there are few data supporting a definitive role of pesticides as a causative factor, but given that only 10% of ALS cases are genetic, a gene-environment cause is likely.[31–33] Pall and colleagues, described a single case report concerning a 59-year-old man who experienced the onset of ALS 2 weeks following high-dose exposure to permethrin.[34] This single case report was followed by another report from Doi and colleagues,[14] reporting the development of motor neuron disease resembling ALS following chronic inhalation of pyrethroid pesticides. Fonseca and colleagues,[35] described 2 Brazilian farmers who worked together, diagnosed with ALS, and demonstrating high blood levels of organochlorine pesticides (aldrin, lindane, heptachlor). Using data from a large case-control study, McGuire and colleagues,[36] found an association between exposure to agricultural chemicals and risk of ALS. However, the odds ratios were relatively low (1.5–2.8). The current data available in the literature suggest that long-term exposures to a variety of pesticides may significantly contribute to neurologic disease. However, much more study is needed with regard to the identification of the specific pesticides that may be involved. In addition, much more study is needed in the emerging area of gene-pesticide interactions with regard to risk for neurologic disease.

REFERENCES

1. Futagami K, Otsubo K, Nakao Y, et al. Acute organophosphate poisoning after disulfoton ingestion. J Toxicol Clin Toxicol 1995;33(2):151–5.
2. Solomon GM, Moodley J. Acute chlorpyrifos poisoning in pregnancy: a case report. Clin Toxicol (Phila) 2007;45(4):416–9.
3. Weiner ML, Jortner BS. Organophosphate-induced delayed neurotoxicity of triarylphosphates. Neurotoxicology 1999;20(4):653–73.
4. Gupta R, editor. Toxicology of organophosphate and carbamate compounds. New York: Elsevier Academic Press; 2006. p. 763.
5. Jett DA, Lein PJ. Non-cholinesterase mechanisms of central and peripheral neurotoxicity: muscarinic receptors and other targets. In: Gupta R, editor. Toxicology of organophosphate and carbamate compounds. New York: Elsevier; 2006. p. 233–46.
6. Hoffman A, Eisenkraft A, Finkelstein A, et al. A decade after the Tokyo sarin attack: a review of neurological follow-up of the victims. Mil Med 2007;172(6): 607–10.
7. Yamasue H, Abe O, Kasai K, et al. Human brain structural change related to acute single exposure to sarin. Ann Neurol 2007;61(1):37–46.
8. Ellenhorn MJ, Schonwald S, Ordog G, et al. Ellenhorn's medical toxicology: diagnosis and treatment of human poisoning. Baltimore (MD): Williams & Wilkins; 1997. p. 1663.
9. Aks SE, Krantz A, Hryhrczuk DO, et al. Acute accidental lindane ingestion in toddlers. Ann Emerg Med 1995;26(5):647–51.
10. Costa LG, Giordano G, Guizzetti M, et al. Neurotoxicity of pesticides: a brief review. Front Biosci 2008;13:1240–9.
11. Safe S. Endocrine disruptors and human health: is there a problem. Toxicology 2004;205(1/2):3–10.
12. Chang LW, Dyer RS. Handbook of neurotoxicology. New York: Marcel Dekker; 1995. p. 1103.
13. Huff JE, Gerstner HB. Kepone: a literature summary. J Environ Pathol Toxicol 1978;1(4):377–95.
14. Doi H, Kikuchi H, Murai H, et al. Motor neuron disorder simulating ALS induced by chronic inhalation of pyrethroid insecticides. Neurology 2006;67(10):1894–5.

15. Power LE, Sudakin DL. Pyrethrin and pyrethroid exposures in the United States: a longitudinal analysis of incidents reported to poison centers. J Med Toxicol 2007;3(3):94–9.
16. Morgan MK, Sheldon LS, Croghan CW, et al. An observational study of 127 preschool children at their homes and daycare centers in Ohio: environmental pathways to cis- and trans-permethrin exposure. Environ Res 2007;104(2):266–74.
17. Kamel F, Hoppin JA. Association of pesticide exposure with neurologic dysfunction and disease. Environ Health Perspect 2004;112(9):950–8.
18. Hatcher JM, Pennell KD, Miller GW. Parkinson's disease and pesticides: a toxicological perspective. Trends Pharmacol Sci 2008;29(6):322–9.
19. Franco R, Li S, Rodriguez-Rocha H, et al. Molecular mechanisms of pesticide-induced neurotoxicity: relevance to Parkinson's disease. Chem Biol Interact 2010;188(2):289–300.
20. Berry C, La Vecchia C, Nicotera P. Paraquat and Parkinson's disease. Cell Death Differ 2010;17(7):1115–25.
21. Fleming L, Mann JB, Bean J, et al. Parkinson's disease and brain levels of organochlorine pesticides. Ann Neurol 1994;36(1):100–3.
22. Corrigan FM, Wienburg CL, Shore RF, et al. Organochlorine insecticides in substantia nigra in Parkinson's disease. J Toxicol Environ Health A 2000;59(4):229–34.
23. Weisskopf MG, Knekt P, O'Reilly EJ, et al. Persistent organochlorine pesticides in serum and risk of Parkinson disease. Neurology 2010;74(13):1055–61.
24. Tanner CM, Ross GW, Jewell SA, et al. Occupation and risk of parkinsonism: a multicenter case-control study. Arch Neurol 2009;66(9):1106–13.
25. Gatto NM, Cockburn M, Bronstein J, et al. Well-water consumption and Parkinson's disease in rural California. Environ Health Perspect 2009;117(12):1912–8.
26. Peng J, Oo ML, Andersen JK. Synergistic effects of environmental risk factors and gene mutations in Parkinson's disease accelerate age-related neurodegeneration. J Neurochem 2010;115(6):1363–73.
27. Benedetto A, Au C, Avila DS, et al. Extracellular dopamine potentiates Mn-induced oxidative stress, lifespan reduction, and dopaminergic neurodegeneration in a BLI-3-dependent manner in Caenorhabditis elegans. PLoS Genet 2010;6(8):e1001084.
28. Santibanez M, Bolumar F, Garcia AM. Occupational risk factors in Alzheimer's disease: a review assessing the quality of published epidemiological studies. Occup Environ Med 2007;64(11):723–32.
29. Baldi I, Lebailly P, Mohammed-Brahim B, et al. Neurodegenerative diseases and exposure to pesticides in the elderly. Am J Epidemiol 2003;157(5):409–14.
30. Hayden KM, Norton MC, Darcey D, et al. Occupational exposure to pesticides increases the risk of incident AD: the Cache County study. Neurology 2010;74(19):1524–30.
31. Johnson FO, Atchison WD. The role of environmental mercury, lead and pesticide exposure in development of amyotrophic lateral sclerosis. Neurotoxicology 2009;30(5):761–5.
32. Morahan JM, Yu B, Trent RJ, et al. Genetic susceptibility to environmental toxicants in ALS. Am J Med Genet B Neuropsychiatr Genet 2007;144B(7):885–90.
33. Qureshi MM, Hayden D, Urbinelli L, et al. Analysis of factors that modify susceptibility and rate of progression in amyotrophic lateral sclerosis (ALS). Amyotroph Lateral Scler 2006;7(3):173–82.
34. Pall HS, Williams AC, Waring R, et al. Motoneurone disease as manifestation of pesticide toxicity. Lancet 1987;2(8560):685.

35. Fonseca RG, Resende LA, Silva MD, et al. Chronic motor neuron disease possibly related to intoxication with organochlorine insecticides. Acta Neurol Scand 1993;88(1):56–8.
36. McGuire V, Longstreth WT Jr, Nelson LM, et al. Occupational exposures and amyotrophic lateral sclerosis. A population-based case-control study. Am J Epidemiol 1997;145(12):1076–88.

Emerging Toxic Neuropathies and Myopathies

Hani A. Kushlaf, MB, BCh

KEYWORDS

- Toxic neuropathies • Toxic myopathies • Myopathy
- Neuropathy

MYOTOXINS
Statins

Statins are a group of drugs used to treat hypercholesterolemia. Approximately 30 million patients use statins in the United States,[1] with approximately 10% of them developing muscle-related complications that range from mild (myalgias) to serious (rhabdomyolysis). Predisposing factors to statin myotoxicity are shown in **Box 1**. Statins have been shown to be associated with several neuromuscular complications,[2] which are summarized in (**Box 2**).

In patients with statin myopathies, muscle biopsies often show nonspecific findings, such as cytochrome oxidase–negative fibers, increased fine lipid droplets, and ragged red fibers.[6]

Although myalgia is reported to develop in approximately 10% of patients taking statins, rhabdomyolysis remains a rare complication. Because diagnostic criteria do not exist for the definition of statin-associated myalgia, this condition is likely an underestimation of the true incidence.

The mechanism of statin-associated myopathy is largely unknown but is thought to be related to impaired prenylation (a process by which hydrophobic groups are added to proteins to facilitate cell membrane binding) of small proteins involved in signal transduction and altered protein glycosylation.[7]

Patients with genetic mutations resulting in either muscular dystrophy or a metabolic myopathy are at a greater risk of developing a statin myopathy. Some patients with *LPIN1* mutation may develop severe myopathy after statin therapy.[8] Single nucleotide polymorphisms on *SLCO1B1*, which encodes the transporter associated with the hepatic uptake of all the statins except fluvastatin, are also associated with increased risk of statin-associated myopathies.[3]

Using statins safely requires regular monitoring for side effects. Specifically, creatine kinase (CK) levels should be measured in all patients before starting a statin.

The author has nothing to disclose.
Department of Neurology, Mayo Clinic, 200 1st Street SW, Rochester, MN 55905, USA
E-mail address: Kushlaf.hani@mayo.edu

Neurol Clin 29 (2011) 679–687
doi:10.1016/j.ncl.2011.05.009
0733-8619/11/$ – see front matter. Published by Elsevier Inc.

Box 1
Risk factors for statin-induced myopathy

Atorvastatin>simvastatin, pravastatin, lovastatin>fluvastatin

Dual therapy with gemfibrozil and a statin

Underlying myopathy (muscular dystrophy, metabolic myopathy, inflammatory myopathy)

Genetic predisposition (eg, SLCO1B1)[3]

Drug-drug interactions (use of cytochrome P450 [CYP3A4] inhibitors, such as verapamil, itraconazole, cyclosporine)

HyperCKemia at baseline suggests an underlying myopathy, and, in these patients, statin treatment has to be monitored cautiously or an alternative medication used. In patients who develop statin-induced myalgia, other causes for myalgias also have to be ruled out, which include fibromyalgia, hypothyroidism, and vitamin D deficiency. Of note, vitamin D deficiency has been shown to increase the risk of statin-induced myalgia.[9]

Asymptomatic hyperCKemia with CK levels less than 3 times normal should be monitored, and the statin drug can be continued. A rising CK level, myoglobinuria, or a CK level higher than ten times the normal level, should prompt immediate statin discontinuation. Discontinuing statin treatment should result in resolution of symptoms, CK normalization, and reversal of muscle biopsy changes within 2 to 3 months.

Patients taking statins can rarely develop an immune-mediated necrotizing myopathy.[10] These patients develop hyperCKemia and proximal muscle weakness, which continue to progress despite statin discontinuation. Although treatment with immunosuppressive agents (eg, steroids and methotrexate) may halt the progression, most patients suffer from some residual weakness.[10] After the statin is discontinued, one may alternatively use a bile acid sequestrant, such as colestipol, or a sterol absorption inhibitor, such as ezetimibe. Other options include using a statin that is less likely to cause a myopathy (eg, fluvastatin) or a statin with a longer half-life every 2 to 3 days instead of daily (eg, atorvastatin); Taking rosuvastatin every other day has been shown to increase its tolerability in patients who were rosuvastatin intolerant with everyday dosing while decreasing their low-density lipoprotein cholesterol levels to a desirable range.[11]

Box 2
Neuromuscular complications described in patients on statins

Myalgia

Asymptomatic hyperCKemia

Acute rhabdomyolysis

Unmasking of other myopathies (eg, mitochondrial myopathy and other metabolic myopathies)

Immune-mediated myopathies

Myasthenia gravis (unmasking or aggravation)[4]

Rippling muscle disease[5]

Peripheral neuropathy

Pharmacogenetic screening does not seem to be cost effective at this point but may become available in the future. In patients with a severe hyperlipidemia who are in need of a fibrate, fenofibrate is a better choice than gemfibrozil because gemfibrozil is known to inhibit CYP2C8 and the hepatic organic anion transporter that are involved in hepatic uptake and metabolism of statins.[12]

Based on epidemiologic studies,[13,14] the incidence of developing a peripheral neuropathy while on a statin is low.

Imatinib Mesylate (Gleevec)

Imatinib is a tyrosine kinase inhibitor used to treat different types of cancer, including gastrointestinal stromal tumors and chronic myeloid leukemia.

In a 2008 case report, a 25-year-old patient receiving 400 mg of imatinib daily for treatment of desmoids tumors temporally developed CK elevations up to 1444 IU/L, with resolution of the hyperCKemia within days after discontinuing the medication.[15] On electromyography, a myopathic pattern was observed in the patient, with the authors concluding that imatinib could cause rhabdomyolysis.[15] After diagnosing rhabdomyolysis in a patient on imatinib, Gordon and colleagues[16] prospectively assessed the 1-year incidence of elevated CK levels in patients on imatinib. Of the 25 patients studied, they found hyperCKemia more than 2 times the upper limit of normal in 20 patients (80%) at some point during their treatment. This finding suggests that myopathy with imatinib may be common and may require routine screening in patients receiving therapy. On the contrary, rhabdomyolysis secondary to imatinib seems to be rare. The mechanism by which imatinib causes myopathy with hyperCKemia is unclear.

Daptomycin

Daptomycin is a lipopeptide antibiotic that works against gram-positive bacteria that has been shown to cause skeletal muscle toxicity in about 1.5% of patients.[17]

Kostrominova and colleagues[18] have shown that scattered muscle fibers are affected in early daptomycin toxicity. The mechanism of toxicity is postulated to be the result of daptomycin integration into the lipid rich outer leaflet of the sarcolemma with resultant calcium influx, which in turn leads to cell death. It is unclear if there is a predisposing factor to daptomycin myotoxicity.

Hydroxychloroquine

Hydroxychloroquine is an aminoquinoline antimalarial agent used for the treatment of connective tissue disorders such as rheumatoid arthritis and systemic lupus erythematosus. Hydroxychloroquine is known to cause mild to moderate vacuolar myopathy, and a recent report suggests that this condition can, at times, be severe and lead to respiratory failure.[19] Abdel-Hamid and colleagues[19] described 2 patients who developed this complication while on hydroxychloroquine. Discontinuing hydroxychloroquine did not improve their weakness. EMG showed positive sharp waves, myotonic discharges, and myopathic motor unit potentials. The CK level was normal in 1 patient and mildy elevated in the other patient. Muscle biopsy results showed fibers harboring rimmed vacuoles, atrophic fibers, and occasional necrotic and regenerating fibers. These rimmed vacuoles showed positive results for acid phosphatase and esterase. The autophagic vacuoles in the muscle biopsies are known features of hydroxychloroquine myotoxicity.

Highly Active Antiretroviral Therapy

Highly active antiretroviral therapy (HAART) is known to be associated with mitochondrial toxicity characterized by fatigue, lactic acidosis, and lipodystrophy.

Pfeffer and colleagues[20] reported on 3 patients who developed a chronic progressive ophthalmoplegia (CPEO) phenotype while on HAART. These patients have been on HAART for 15 to 18 years. One patient had an underlying mitochondrial DNA deletion, which was thought to be subclinical, and the patient expressed the CPEO phenotype after exposure to HAART. This patient had a levator palpebrae superioris biopsy during a procedure for ptosis that showed an abundance of ragged red fibers and cytochrome C oxidase (COX)-negative fibers. A quadriceps muscle biopsy in the same patient showed subsarcolemmal increases of oxidative enzyme activity and some COX-negative fibers. To further support the hypothesis of causation, the symptoms of one patient (fatigue, headache, and ptosis) improved after cessation of HAART.[20]

This report demonstrates that patients who present with a mitochondrial disease phenotype including CPEO, indeed, may have an underlying mitochondrial disease that became manifest with the use of mitochondrial toxic drugs.

NEUROMUSCULAR JUNCTION TOXINS
Tandutinib

Tandutinib (MLN 518, Millennium Pharmaceuticals, Cambridge, MA, USA) is a tyrosine kinase inhibitor currently in clinical trials for the treatment of glioblastoma multiforme. In one study[15] of 40 patients received a combination of tandutinib and bevacizumab, 6 developed muscle weakness. These patients developed facial weakness, neck weakness, and proximal greater than distal limb weakness. None of the patients developed ocular or pharyngeal weakness. Two patients had to discontinue the medication because of the weakness, even at a lower dose, whereas, 4 patients were able to tolerate the medication at lower doses. Repetitive nerve stimulation (RNS) showed a decremental response in patients evaluated with RNS, and, in 1 patient, improvement was shown after 1 week of drug discontinuation. Single-fiber EMG showed abnormal jitter with blocking in patients evaluated with single-fiber EMG.[21]

The mechanism of tandutinib neuromuscular junction toxicity is unclear, and studies are needed to clarify the pathophysiology underlying tandutinib toxic effect.

PERIPHERAL NERVE TOXINS
Bortezomib

Bortezomib (Velcade) is a selective 26S proteasome inhibitor used for the treatment of multiple myeloma and refractory or relapsed mantle cell lymphoma. Bortezomib is known to cause peripheral neuropathy that is mostly distal, sensory, and length dependent. In a study by Chaudhry and colleagues,[22] some patients developed a reversible demyelinating neuropathy and other patients developed perioral and scalp paresthesias, arguing for a sensory ganglionopathy as a possible site of toxicity. A single patient was reported to have an inflammatory neuropathy based on nerve biopsy findings and improvement on dexamethasone.[23] Cases of severe motor neuropathy have also been reported with bortezomib. In a cell culture study by Watanabe and colleagues,[24] the investigators demonstrated that compounds that induce heat shock protein 70 or lysosomal-associated membrane protein 2A are expected to improve or prevent bortezomib-induced peripheral neuropathy. Future clinical trials with the previously mentioned compounds are required to confirm and test this observation.

At present, the treatment is supportive with the treatment of neuropathic pain and use of orthoses. The sensory symptoms may improve as in the neuropathy caused by other chemotherapeutic agents.

Angel's Trumpet

Ingestion of angel's trumpet flowers (*Brugmansia suaveolens*; syn *Datura suaveolens*) is recently reported to cause the acute motor axonal neuropathy variant of Guillain-Barré syndrome.

In one case report, a 5-year-old boy developed a generalized weakness with difficulty in breathing, in addition to a left tonic pupil, after allegedly eating white flowers from the backyard.[25] Physical examination showed that the patient was generally weak, had generalized hyporeflexia, and had tachypnea (60 per minute). Magnetic resonance imaging (MRI) of the lumbar spine showed enhancement of the nerve roots of the cauda equina. Cerebrospinal fluid (CSF) analysis showed a cell count of 11, a protein level of 70 mg/dL, and a glucose level of 100 mg/dL. The patient did not respond to intravenous immunoglobulin (IVIG) and plasmaphresis. After recovery in 45 days, the patient reported eating white flowers from the backyard.

The mechanism by which angel trumpet causes Guillain-Barré is unclear; however, it could be related to an aberrant immune response similar to that seen after a variety of infections (Epstein-Barr virus, cytomegalovirus, hepatitis, varicella, and other herpes viruses, *Mycoplasma pneumoniae*, and *Campylobacter jejuni*), as well as immunizations that have been known to precede or to be associated with the illness. Angel's trumpet is in the nightshade family; it contains the alkaloids atropine, hyoscine, and scopolamine in a relatively high concentration, which makes it highly toxic. The predominant toxic syndrome seen in clinical practice is an anticholinergic syndrome. Unilateral tonic pupil has been reported in angel's trumpet intoxications.[26]

Because this is a single case report from a suspected ingestion, the association between angel's trumpet and the development of neuropathy is not clear at this time. It may be important to consider inquiring about plant ingestions in addition to tick paralysis when faced with a Guillain-Barré–like syndrome in a child.

Cisplatin

Cisplatin is a platinum-based antineoplastic alkylating agent used for the treatment of several cancers. It is well known that cisplatin causes chemotherapy-related peripheral neuropathy[27]; 90% of patients receiving a cumulative dose of 300 mg/m^2 or more develop a peripheral neuropathy. Recently, vitamin E was tried in a double-blind placebo-controlled trial to evaluate its neuroprotective effect.[28] A total of 108 patients receiving more than 300 mg/m^2 of cisplatin were randomized to vitamin E (400 mg/d) or placebo. The incidence of neurotoxicity was significantly lower in the vitamin E group (5.9%) compared with the placebo group (41.7%) ($P = .01$), demonstrating the potential effectiveness of vitamin E in preventing the neurotoxic effects of cisplatin.[28]

Oxaliplatin

Oxaliplatin is another platinum-based drug similar to cisplatin. Oxaliplatin causes a chronic sensory neurotoxicity similar to cisplatin, but it is also shown to cause acute motor nerve hyperexcitability that seems to be mechanistically different.[29] Hill and colleagues[30] demonstrated this phenomenon using motor nerve conduction studies and needle EMG. Repetitive compound motor action potentials were seen in 71% of patients. Abnormal high-frequency spontaneous motor fiber action potentials were seen in 100% of patients on days 2 to 4 after oxaliplatin treatment and decreased in frequency to 25% on days 14 to 20 after oxaliplatin treatment. The neuropathy induced by oxaliplatin seems to be long term and does not reverse completely on discontinuation.[31]

Tacrolimus

Tacrolimus is a potent immunosuppressant used to prevent organ transplant rejections (heart, kidney, and liver).

A recent case report showed that tacrolimus causes a toxic optic neuropathy. The frequency of this adverse effect seems to be rare.[32] The patient had undergone cardiac and renal transplants and developed asynchronous visual loss after taking tacrolimus for 5 years. MRI of the brain showed an optic nerve enlargement. Optic nerve biopsy showed evidence of demyelination without evidence of vasculitis. The patient did not improve after discontinuation of tacrolimus, which may indicate the irreversibility of this adverse effect. The investigators claimed that this report was the first report of toxic demyelination because most toxic agents cause axonopathies; however, it is unclear from the published report whether the demyelination is secondary to an axonal pathology and is clustered or primary, hence the need for teased fiber preparation to be done to differentiate between the two. The author argues that demyelination is secondary in this patient because the report showed endoneurial and perivascular macrophages in addition to axonal degeneration. The presence of these findings makes axonal degeneration the likely explanation of the observed demyelination.

Tumor Necrosis Factor α Antagonists

Tumor necrosis factor α (TNF-α) antagonists are important immunomodulators used for the treatment of several rheumatologic conditions, including rheumatoid arthritis, ankylosing spondylitis, psoriatic arthritis, Crohn disease, and ulcerative colitis. TNF-α antagonists include etanercept, infliximab, and adalimumab.

There are several reports associating the use of TNF-α antagonists with Guillain-Barré syndrome, Miller Fisher syndrome, chronic inflammatory demyelinating polyneuropathy, multifocal motor neuropathy with conduction block, mononeuropathy multiplex, and axonal sensorimotor polyneuropathies.[33]

Alshekhlee and colleagues[34] reported on 2 patients who developed chronic idiopathic demyelinating polyneuropathy while on treatment with etanercept and infliximab, respectively. The onset of symptoms varied between 2 weeks and 12 months of treatment with TNF-α antagonists. The mechanism of immune-mediated neuropathies in patients treated with TNF-α is unclear and remains to be fully explained. In contrast to previous reports, these 2 patients became dependent on immunosuppressive therapy instead of improvement on withdrawal of TNF-α antagonists.[34] Careful monitoring of patients is necessary to be aware of these immune-mediated neuropathies at an early stage during treatment with TNF-α antagonists.

Cobalt-Chromium

Ikeda and colleagues[35] reported on a patient who underwent a hip arthroplasty (cobalt-chromium prosthesis) 5 years before the development of symptoms. The symptoms consisted of gait disturbance, dysesthesias in all extremities, and auditory difficulties. The patient also had bilateral sensorineural hearing loss, which has been reported in patients with cobalt toxicity.[36]

Blood and sural nerve levels of cobalt and chromium were elevated and decreased after a revision surgery with ceramic-on-ceramic prosthesis; revision was also associated with improvement in symptoms. EMG showed absent sensory responses on nerve conduction studies. All motor responses were normal in nerve conduction studies. No needle examination was reported in the study.[35] A sural nerve biopsy showed decreased myelinated fiber density with a selective loss of large myelinated fibers. No significant inflammation was found. The findings on biopsy are in keeping with an axonal neuropathy. Sensory impairment in patients with artificial joints should raise a suspicion of this condition.

Zinc

Zinc is used in denture creams. Zinc induces intestinal metallothionein, which preferentially binds copper and is lost in feces with sloughed enterocytes. Hyperzincemia is shown in a study by Nations and colleagues[37] to be associated with hypocupremic myeloneuropathy. Myelopathy presents with spastic paraparesis, ataxia, and impairment of dorsal column sensations. The peripheral neuropathy tends to be sensory predominant and can be painful. Motor neuron disease–like presentation can occur in the setting of hypocupremia. Spinazzi and colleagues[38] questioned hyperzincemia as the sole cause of hypocupremia and pointed out that most patients with hypocupremic myeloneuropathy have other contributing factors, such as gastrointestinal surgeries, malnutrition, or malabsorption syndromes. A workup to exclude such factors is necessary in patients with hypocupremic myeloneuropathy. Discontinuing the use of zinc-based denture creams results in improvement of the hypocupremia and stabilization or mild improvement of the syndrome.

Ixabepilone

Ixabepilone is an epothilone B analogue that works as a microtubule stabilizer and is approved for use in the treatment of metastatic or locally advanced breast cancer (refractory or resistant). The most common adverse effects of ixabepilone are neutropenia and peripheral neuropathy.[39] The peripheral neuropathy is primarily sensory, is dose dependent, and reverses on discontinuation. The median time to improvement in symptoms is 4 to 6 weeks. Significant neuropathy usually develops after the third or fourth cycle of treatment. Depending on the severity of the neuropathy, lowering the dose may suffice in some patients.

Porcine Neural Tissue

Lachance and colleagues[40] reported on 24 patients who were exposed to aerosolized porcine neural tissue while working in 2 different swine abattoirs. A total of 21 patients developed an inflammatory painful sensory-predominant polyradiculoneuropathy with mild dysautonomia at the onset. The presentations included difficulty in walking, fatigue, sensory disturbances with burning, and aching pains. More than half the patients had an associated headache. Three patients developed aseptic meningitis, transverse myelitis, and meningoencephalitis, which were followed by a painful polyradiculoneuropathy. CSF analysis showed elevated CSF protein level in 18 of 21 tested patients and a pleocytosis in 3 of 21 tested patients. There was a preferential involvement of areas lacking in blood-brain barrier in all patients, such as dorsal root ganglia, dorsal roots, and distal sensory and motor nerves. The proximal involvement was identified on eliciting pain consistently with root stretching maneuvers, nerve conduction studies showing prolonged F-wave latencies and trigeminal blink responses, a thermoregulatory sweat testing showing a polyradicular pattern of sweat loss, and MRI showing enlargement and enhancement of nerve roots and ganglia. The involvement of distal sensory and motor nerves was identified on nerve conduction studies showing prolonged distal motor and sensory latencies, distal sweat loss on thermoregulatory sweat testing, and distal abnormalities on quantitative sensory testing. Sural nerve biopsies in 4 patients showed findings of inflammatory demyelination. Seventeen of the patients underwent treatment with immunosuppressive agents including intravenous methylprednisolone, IVIG, plasma exchange, and oral prednisone resulting in improvement in motor symptoms; however, most patients were left with residual pain and sensory symptoms. Autoimmunity developing after exposure to porcine neural tissue was suspected to be the cause of this syndrome.

SUMMARY

This article described new, and potentially new, toxic myopathies, neuropathies, and neuromuscular junction syndromes. Of the toxins discussed, there is little consensus as to the prevention or treatment of toxicity. In addition, the mechanism of toxicity or causation in many of the identified peripheral nerve toxins is still unclear. The identification of new toxic syndromes requires careful analysis of the clinical presentation of patients, in addition to paying close attention to demographic and occupational attributes. Further research is required to further elucidate the basic mechanisms underlying these toxic syndromes, thus identifying plans for prevention and treatment.

REFERENCES

1. Stagniti MN. Trends in statins utilization and expenditure for the U.S. civilian noninstitutionalized population, 2000 and 2005. Agency for Healthcare Research and Quality. Statistical brief #205, May 2008.
2. Mastalgia FL. Iatrogenic myopathies. Curr Opin Neurol 2010;23:445–9.
3. Link E, Parish S, Armitage J, et al. SLCO1B1 variants and statin-induced myopathy—a genome wide study. N Engl J Med 2008;359:789–99.
4. Purvin V, Kawasaki A, Smith KH, et al. Statin-associated myasthenia gravis: report of 4 cases and review of the literature. Medicine 2006;85:82–5.
5. Baker SK, Tarnopolsky MA. Sporadic rippling muscle disease unmasked by simvastatin. Muscle Nerve 2006;34:478–81.
6. Oskarsson B. Myopathy: five new things. Neurology 2011;76:S14.
7. Vaklavas C, Chatzizisis YS, Ziakas A, et al. Molecular basis of statin-associated myopathy. Atherosclerosis 2009;202:18–28.
8. Zeharia A, Shaag A, Houtkooper RH, et al. Mutations in LPIN1 cause recurrent acute myoglobinuria in childhood. Am J Hum Genet 2008;83:489–94.
9. Lee P, Greenfield JR, Campbell LV. Vitamin D insufficiency—a novel mechanism of statin-induced myalgia? Clin Endocrinol (Oxf) 2009;71:154–5.
10. Grable-Esposito P, Katzberg HD, Greenberg SA, et al. Immune-mediated necrotizing myopathy associated with statins. Muscle Nerve 2010;41:185–90.
11. Backes JM, Venero CV, Gibson CA, et al. Effectiveness and tolerability of every-other-day rosuvastatin dosing in patients with prior statin intolerance. Ann Pharmacother 2008;42:341–6.
12. Neuvonen PJ, Niemi M, Backman JT. Drug interactions with lipid-lowering drugs: mechanisms and clinical relevance. Clin Pharmacol Ther 2006;80:565–81.
13. Lovastatin Study Groups I Through IV. Lovastatin 5-year safety and efficacy study. Arch Intern Med 1993;153:1079–87.
14. Gaist D, Jeppesen U, Andersen M, et al. Statins and risk of polyneuropathy: a case-control study. Neurology 2002;58:1333–7.
15. Penel N, Blay JY, Adenis A. Imatinib as a possible cause of rhabdomyolysis. N Engl J Med 2008;358:2746–7.
16. Gordon JK, Magid SK, Makib RG, et al. Elevations of creatine kinase in patients treated with imatinib mesylate. Leuk Res 2010;34:827–9.
17. Rybak MJ. The efficacy and safety of daptomycin: first in a new class of antibiotics for Gram-positive bacteria. Clin Microbiol Infect 2006;12(Suppl 1):24–32.

18. Kostrominova TY, Hassett CA, Rader EP, et al. Characterization of skeletal muscle effects associated with daptomycin in rats. Muscle Nerve 2010;42:385–93.

19. Abdel-Hamid H, Oddis CV, Lacomis D. Severe hydroxychloroquine myopathy. Muscle Nerve 2008;38:1206–10.

20. Pfeffer G, Côté HC, Montaner JS, et al. Ophthalmoplegia and ptosis: mitochondrial toxicity in patients receiving HIV therapy. Neurology 2009;73:71–2.

21. Lehky TJ, Iwamoto FM, Kreisl TN, et al. Neuromuscular junction toxicity with tandutinib induces a myasthenic-like syndrome. Neurology 2011;76:236–41.

22. Chaudhry V, Cornblath DR, Polydefkis M, et al. Characteristics of bortezomib- and thalidomide-induced peripheral neuropathy. J Peripher Nerv Syst 2008;13:275–82.

23. Saifee TA, Elliott KJ, Lunn MP, et al. Bortezomib-induced inflammatory neuropathy. J Peripher Nerv Syst 2010;15:366–8.

24. Watanabe T, Nagase K, Chosa M, et al. Schwann cell autophagy induced by SAHA, 17 AAG, or clonazepam can reduce bortezomib-induced peripheral neuropathy. Br J Cancer 2010;103:1580–7.

25. Sevketoglu E, Tatli B, Tuğcu B, et al. An unusual cause of fulminant Guillain-Barré syndrome: angel's trumpet. Pediatr Neurol 2010;43:368–70.

26. Andriol B, Povan A, Da Dolt L, et al. Unilateral mydriasis due to angel's trumpet. Clin Toxicol 2008;46:329–31.

27. Alberts DS, Noel JK. Cisplatin-associated neurotoxicity: can it be prevented? Anticancer Drugs 1995;6:369–83.

28. Pace A, Giannarelli D, Galiè E, et al. Vitamin E neuroprotection for cisplatin neuropathy: a randomized, placebo-controlled trial. Neurology 2010;74:762–6.

29. Lehky TJ, Leonard GD, Wilson RH, et al. Oxaliplatin-induced neurotoxicity: acute hyperexcitability and chronic neuropathy. Muscle Nerve 2004;29:387–92.

30. Hill A, Bergin P, Hanning F, et al. Detecting acute neurotoxicity during platinum chemotherapy by neurophysiological assessment of motor nerve Hyperexcitability. BMC Cancer 2010;10:451.

31. Park SB, Lin CS, Krishnan AV, et al. Long-term neuropathy after oxaliplatin treatment: challenging the dictum of reversibility. Oncologist 2011;16(5):708–16.

32. Venneti S, Moss HE, Levin MH, et al. Asymmetric bilateral demyelinating optic neuropathy from tacrolimus toxicity. J Neurol Sci 2011;301:112–5.

33. Stübgen JP. Tumor necrosis factor-alpha antagonists and neuropathy. Muscle Nerve 2008;37:281–92.

34. Alshekhlee A, Basiri K, Miles JD, et al. Chronic inflammatory demyelinating polyneuropathy associated with TNF-α antagonists. Muscle Nerve 2010;41:732–7.

35. Ikeda T, Takahashi K, Kabata T, et al. Polyneuropathy caused by cobalt-chromium metallosis after total hip replacement. Muscle Nerve 2010;42:140–3.

36. Oldenburg M, Wegner R, Baur X. Severe cobalt intoxication due to prosthesis wear in repeated total hip arthroplasty. J Arthroplasty 2009;24:825.e15–20.

37. Nations SP, Boyer PJ, Love LA, et al. Denture cream: an unusual source of excess zinc, leading to hypocupremia and neurologic disease. Neurology 2008;71:639–43.

38. Spinazzi M, De Lazzari F, Tavolato B, et al. Myelo-opticoneuropathy in copper deficiency occurring after partial gastrectomy: do small bowel bacterial overgrowth syndrome and occult zinc ingestion tip the balance? J Neurol 2007;254:1012–7.

39. Yardley DA. Proactive management of adverse events maintains the clinical benefit of ixabepilone. Oncologist 2009;14:448–55.

40. Lachance DH, Lennon VA, Pittock SJ, et al. An outbreak of neurological autoimmunity with polyradiculoneuropathy in workers exposed to aerosolized porcine neural tissue: a descriptive study. Lancet Neurol 2010;9:55–66.

Amyotrophic Lateral Sclerosis: What Role Does Environment Play?

Aiesha Ahmed, MD, Matthew P. Wicklund, MD*

KEYWORDS

- Amyotrophic lateral sclerosis • Environment
- Motor neuron disease • Toxin

DISEASE OVERVIEW

Amyotrophic lateral sclerosis (ALS) is a disorder of progressive upper and lower motor neuron degeneration and was initially described by Charcot in 1874.[1] Lower motor neuron loss manifests as weakness, muscular atrophy, and fasciculations, whereas brisk muscle stretch reflexes, clonus, motor dyscontrol, and Babinski signs reflect upper motor neuron disease. Sensory and autonomic systems are spared. Now the evidence also suggests frontal executive deficits in half of patients with ALS and frank frontotemporal lobar dementia in a smaller segment.[2] Disease onset occurs roughly equally in the bulbar, cervical, and lumbar regions, with death ensuing in 1 to 6 years.[3] Death occurs most often because of respiratory failure. Prognosis for survival in bulbar onset ALS is much shorter than for ALS with initial lower extremity onset. Isolated lower motor neuron involvement is called progressive muscular atrophy (PMA), whereas strictly upper motor neuron disease is called primary lateral sclerosis (PLS). Both PMA and PLS advance more slowly, but often ultimately transform into ALS.

The incidence and prevalence of ALS increase with age through the seventh to eighth decade, with men suffering the disorder roughly twice as frequently as women. Epidemiologic studies suggest an increasing incidence of ALS over time. However, this observed increase likely relates to aging of the world's population, greater precision in diagnosis of ALS, and better case ascertainment.[4] Worldwide, incidence rates of 0.6 to 2.6 per 100,000 and prevalence rates of 1.5 to 8.5 per 100,000 occur nearly

The views expressed herein are those of the authors. The authors have no external sources of funding to report.

Department of Neurology, Hershey Medical Center, Penn State Milton South, 30 Hope Drive - EC037, Hershey, PA 17033, USA

* Corresponding author.

E-mail address: mwicklund@hmc.psu.edu

Neurol Clin 29 (2011) 689–711
doi:10.1016/j.ncl.2011.06.001
0733-8619/11/$ – see front matter © 2011 Elsevier Inc. All rights reserved.

uniformly across the globe,[5] with a lifetime likelihood of mortality from ALS of roughly 1:1000. More patients with ALS seem to be born in the spring months. Isolated regions in the western Pacific including Guam, the Kii Peninsula of Japan, and western New Guinea have had markedly increased incidence rates in the past, sparking research of these populations.

Diagnosis of ALS requires demonstration of both upper and lower motor neuron dysfunction. Other neurologic systems tend not be affected, and ALS mimickers must be excluded.[6,7] World Federation of Neurology El Escorial criteria for a diagnosis of definite ALS require evidence for upper and lower motor neuron disease in 3 of 4 regions (bulbar, cervical, thoracic, lumbar). Newer electrodiagnostic criteria, the Awaji criteria, augment the importance of clinical features and incorporate fasciculation potentials into this diagnostic algorithm.[8] The Awaji criteria may allow increased sensitivity and earlier diagnosis without sacrificing diagnostic specificity.[9] Abnormalities in magnetic resonance imaging, magnetic resonance spectroscopy, magnetic resonance diffusion tensor imaging, and cortical magnetic stimulation may document disease in upper motor neurons.[10,11] Electromyography confirms the lower motor neuron dysfunction in addition to quantifying the number of remaining motor neurons.[12] Although readily diagnosed clinically, the differential diagnosis of ALS remains broad. Diagnostic considerations to exclude include hyperthyroidism, hyperparathyroidism, brainstem disease, intrinsic and extrinsic disease of the cervical spinal cord, Kennedy disease, Hirayama disease, postpolio syndrome, hexosaminidase deficiency, polyradiculopathies and myeloradiculopathies, multifocal motor neuropathy, neuromuscular junction disorders, and inflammatory myopathies.[13] Serology, electromyography, neuroimaging, and mutation analysis exclude these alternative diagnoses.

At the current time, treatment options for ALS remain limited and mostly ineffective. Riluzole, a glutamate antagonist, is the only agent on the market documented to affect disease progression in ALS. In the published trial, the time to death or respiratory failure (a surrogate marker for death) in the treatment group was 18 months as opposed to 15 months in the placebo group, a benefit of 3 additional months of life.[14] Most patients in this trial had moderately advanced disease, and it is believed that treatment early in the course provides up to a year's benefit in life extension. Many patients are also treated with other agents such as antioxidants, coenzyme Q10, creatine, and multiple other agents with hopes that these may benefit survival. Lamotrigene, gabapentin, dextromethorphan, selegiline, brain-derived neurotrophic factor, insulinlike growth factor, glial-derived growth factor, cyclophosphamide, levamisole, amantadine, and lithium have all proved ineffective in controlled clinical trials.

Although most ALS cases occur sporadically, roughly 10% are familial.[15] In 1993, mutations were first reported in the gene for copper/zinc superoxide dismutase (SOD1), which catalyzes dismutation of the superoxide radical to hydrogen peroxide and oxygen.[16] More than 100 different SOD1 mutations have since been discovered.[17–19] Most SOD1 mutations follow autosomal dominant inheritance. However, some recessive ALS families carry homozygous D90A mutations in the SOD1 gene.[20] Initially, SOD1 mutations were believed to exert deleterious effects by decreased enzymatic activity leading to excitotoxicity. However, it is now believed that SOD1 enzyme activity does not correlate with disease expression,[21] and SOD1 knockout mouse models do not develop ALS.[22] Dominant SOD1 mutations are considered to act via a toxic gain of function caused by accumulation of abnormal SOD1 protein products.[18] Genetic testing in sporadic ALS cases estimates that ~10% of these cases also carry a genetic underpinning.[23,24] More than 20 chromosomal loci are now known to underlie different genetic forms of ALS with gene products delineated in at least 15.[19,25]

Because of low incidence and prevalence rates, large, randomized, prospective cohort studies are difficult to perform in ALS. Much research into the cause of ALS has therefore been conducted with case-control studies in the past several decades.

Case-control studies allow evaluation of putative risk factors for disease by retrospectively comparing their presence or absence in patients and matched controls. Patient and control selection and data collection methodology may lead to multiple sources of bias. Some forms of bias unfairly favor the hypothesis and others decrease its likelihood. Case-control studies also identify only associations, not necessarily causal relationships. Selection bias may lead to patient populations derived from samples not reflective of the disease population (eg, patients with ALS referred to a university hospital's neuromuscular center tend to be younger and more atypical in presentation). Nonrespondent bias may unwittingly exclude key portions of the patient or control populations. Inversely, overmatching of patient and control populations might diminish the chance of finding a difference between 2 populations (eg, patients and controls from the same workplace or households might have similar exposures). Recall bias is difficult to exclude. Patients more commonly recall exposures, whereas controls, with less at stake, more often do not. Interviewers not blinded to the patient's condition (challenging with infirm patients with ALS with disabilities) may inadvertently probe harder for details from patients than from controls (interviewer bias). An inadequate sample size reduces a study's statistical power and constrains the possibility of delineating small, but key, differences between groups. If the cause of ALS is multifactorial, small differences in only a portion of a population may be diluted and not detected. Multiple statistical determinations increase the likelihood of finding 1 or more associations based solely on chance. Even with all these limitations, case-control studies still supply the bulwark of data comprising our knowledge of putative ALS risk factors.

HEAVY METALS AND TRACE ELEMENTS

Because of clinical similarities between some heavy metal poisoning cases and ALS, and also because of the correlation of certain trace elements with clusters of motor neuron disease, early importance was placed on investigation of these factors. Callaghan and colleagues[26] reviewed the relevant literature regarding metal exposures and the risk of developing ALS and found that many different metals have been implicated in ALS. However, metals either have inconclusive, conflicting, or insufficient results to make a definitive conclusion. One explanation for these findings is that metal exposures alone are insufficient for the development of ALS. Perhaps an interaction between the metal exposure and an individual's genetic makeup is required to produce epigenetic changes ultimately leading to ALS.

Lead

As early as 1907,[27] through to now,[28] toxicity caused by lead poisoning has been known to cause a motor polyneuropathy sometimes mimicking ALS.[29,30] Numerous case-control studies evaluated lead's role in ALS. Several of these studies purport a greater association with lead exposure for patients than for controls,[31-36] whereas other studies fail to find such an association.[37-39] Investigators also found increased concentrations of lead in cerebrospinal fluid,[40,41] plasma,[42] blood,[36] skeletal muscle,[43,44] nerve,[44] spinal cord,[44,45] and bone.[36] The significance of lead accumulation in these tissues in ALS is of uncertain causal significance. Mandybur and Cooper[46] elegantly showed that accumulation of spinal cord lead content was independent of lead intake in rats with experimental allergic encephalitis (EAE). Spinal cords in diseased rats with EAE (whether or not fed a diet high in lead) accumulated twice the lead concentration as control rats. They concluded that lead accumulation in spinal cords might be a manifestation of disease and not of lead intake or exposure. Other investigators found no difference in lead levels in blood[47,48] or toenails (a good source for evaluation of exposures in the past 6–18 months).[49] Chelation therapy leads to clinical improvement in patients with lead-associated motor polyneuropathies.[29] However, this treatment modality provides no benefit in sporadic ALS.[50–52] Based on the Callaghan and colleagues[26] review, despite many studies, the role, if any, of this metal in the pathogenesis of ALS still remains unclear. Lead toxicity may cause a syndrome with features of ALS but, without other symptoms of lead toxicity or a history of lead exposure, testing or treating for lead toxicity is not warranted. There does not seem to be a strong association between lead and the development of ALS.

Mercury

Analogous to lead, acute and chronic mercury poisoning spawn ALS-like syndromes. This association has been known for the past half century,[53–56] and reports of this association continue.[57] Two case-control studies discovered that more patients with ALS report exposure to mercury than controls,[31,32] and another case-control study found greater job exposure to arsenic, manganese, mercury, or other heavy metals.[33] Heavy metal exposure was not more common in patients with ALS in 3 case-control studies.[37,38,58] Many humans seem to accumulate mercury in spinal motor neurons by late adulthood, but no difference was found between spinal cords from patients with ALS and controls.[59] Mercury concentrations in blood, plasma, and red blood cells were not different from controls.[48] Unless chronic or acute exposure to mercury is noted on clinical grounds, screening for mercury seems without merit.

Aluminum

In the middle of the last century, reports of ALS incidence rates 50-fold to 100-fold higher than elsewhere in the world were noted in the western Pacific. High prevalence rates of a parkinsonism-dementia complex (PDC) also intermingled in these populations. The resultant disease was called Guamanian or western Pacific ALS-PDC. Epidemiologic studies uncovered low amounts of Ca and Mg along with high amounts of Al and Mn in the soil and drinking water from these regions.[60,61] Al has been detected in neurofibrillary tangles in brains of patients with ALS-PDC.[62] Cynomolgus monkeys fed low-Ca/Mg and high-Al diets have exhibited intraneuronal aluminum accumulation along with neuronal loss consistent with ALS.[63] Intracisternal injection of aluminum in animal models leads to a clinical ALS phenotype with motor neuron loss.[64–66] Mice chronically fed low-Ca/Mg and high-Al diets show degeneration and reduction in neuronal numbers in spinal cord and cerebral cortex[67] along with typical skin changes associated with ALS.[68] Low dietary Ca and Mg increase intestinal absorption of Al. Excessive environmental exposure to aluminum was not confirmed in a recent case-control study.[49] Aluminum may play a role in development of motor neuron disease as a sole agent in some patients or as a contributing factor in patients. There are plausible biologic data using animal models suggesting deleterious effects of aluminum on motor neurons, perhaps enhanced by dietary factors.

Selenium

Kilness and Hochberg[69] observed a cluster of ALS cases in a high-Se environment in 1976. Kurlander and Patten[45] then documented a higher spinal cord Se concentration in a single patient compared with 3 controls. Subsequently, Se levels were found to be increased in blood, spinal cord, liver, and bone of patients with ALS.[70,71] An Italian case-control study described a high incidence of ALS in a population exposed to drinking water with a high Se content.[72] Recent studies have not replicated findings of increased blood Se levels in patients with ALS nor accumulation of Se in their toenails.[47–49] As with most other heavy metals, Se may play a role in the pathogenesis of motor neuron disease; however, strong epidemiologic evidence remains lacking.

Manganese

Occupational Mn exposure causing a parkinsonian syndrome was first reported in the 1800s. It has been well studied since then.[73] Extrapolating the concept that Mn causes one neurodegenerative disorder, increased Mn levels in spinal cords of patients with ALS were reported.[45,71] Mn concentrations in blood cells from patients with ALS are significantly lower than in disease controls and healthy people.[70] Case-control studies do not suggest increased occupational exposure to Mn for patients with ALS.[58] Recent studies failed to document accumulation of Mn in blood or toenails.[48,49] Manganese superoxide dismutase (SOD2) is the mitochondrial isoenzyme inactivating superoxide radicals and a cousin to cytosolic Cu/Zn SOD1. This sole difference between mitochondrial and cytosolic superoxide dismutase spurs curiosity into the pathogenesis of Mn. Thus far, no disease-causing mutations have been found in the SOD2 gene.[74]

Other Metals and Trace Elements

Pamphlett and colleagues[48] published an evaluation of cadmium, lead, mercury, copper, zinc, selenium, and manganese blood levels from 20 patients with ALS and an equal number of partner controls. Cd levels were statistically increased in patients with ALS versus controls but with considerable overlap in their values. Copper and zinc are integral components of Cu/Zn cytosolic superoxide dismutase (SOD1). Finding mutations in the SOD1 gene sparked curiosity into levels of these elements in ALS.[75] Bromine, zinc, rubidium, and iron concentrations in erythrocytes were not different between disease and control groups.[70] Magnesium, chromium, iron, cobalt, zinc, rubidium, cesium, antimony, silver, and copper levels in ALS spinal cord samples did not differ from control spinal cord levels.[71] Using toenail clippings as biomarkers of chronic exposure, concentrations of copper, chromium, cobalt, and iron in 22 patients revealed no differences compared with 40 controls.[49]

TOXINS/CHEMICALS/SOLVENTS

The incidence of ALS in the western Pacific region was far higher than elsewhere worldwide and remains increased today. Therefore, reports of clusters of ALS cases in a particular household, geographic location, workplace, or occupation promote speculation concerning common environmental factors afflicting particular populations or geographic locales. Both a husband and wife may develop ALS. Because reports of conjugal ALS remain rare, this occurrence probably reflects the combined odds of both older persons in a marriage developing the same uncommon disease.[76,77] Published reports of clusters in the United States have not always been shown by further statistical evaluation to exceed endemic incidence rates.[78–80] A prospective study in the United Kingdom did find a low background incidence of ALS studded with pockets of higher incidence.[81] These investigators postulate the geographic distribution of ALS to be nonrandom. Mendell and colleagues[82] published the cases of 3 teachers developing ALS. All 3 taught in the same classroom at an Ohio high school. None had other common exposures in terms of the locations of their homes, hobbies, dietary habits, medications, or family history of neurologic disease. They were not interrelated. An investigation of the school yielded no toxic source. Statistical analysis determined the probability of these 3 teachers in that school developing ALS to be very low (P<.0001) and the probability of any 3 teachers dying from ALS at any of Ohio's 878 schools was also low (P<.05).[82] One large, suspected occupational cluster associated with employment at an Air Force base in Texas was evaluated with a mortality ascertainment study. Using death certificates, investigators found that mortality from motor neuron disease and, in particular, ALS, was not increased in this population compared with statewide ALS death rates. The investigators plan to reinvestigate this population again 10 years later because of the potential long latency from toxic exposure to death from ALS.[83] With the advent of genetic techniques, some apparent geographic clusters of sporadic ALS are now discovered to be caused by a common genetic defect, likely from a common ancestor.[84]

Farming

The pathogenic mechanisms by which employment in the agricultural sector might lead to ALS relate to chemical exposures (fertilizers, insecticides, herbicides), exposures to animals and their associated diseases, or the physical nature of the work. In 1977, Rosati and colleagues[85] observed an association between employment in farming and an increased risk of ALS in Sardinia, in southern Italy. These findings have been expanded for the Sardinia region[86] and replicated in the province of Ferrara, in northern Italy.[38] In the northern Italian study, a significant association was found for farmers and persons living in rural areas, but not for work with agricultural chemicals. Another Italian case-control study with more than 500 patients with ALS and controls found greater numbers of farmers and an overabundance of exposure to chemical products in patients.[87] A large case-control study out of western Washington State in the United States comparing 174 patients with 348 age-matched and sex-matched controls provided further evidence for an association between agricultural employment and ALS. This blinded, population-based study derived its control patients mostly via random-digit dialing, a method minimizing common geographic or occupational exposures. Although the odds ratio (OR) was not robust (OR, 2.0, with 95% confidence intervals [CI] of 1.1–3.5), the narrow confidence window adds to this finding's strength.[39] The findings pertained only to men and not to women, but did show a dose-response relationship. Men with the highest exposure rates to agricultural chemicals suffered the highest ORs. Other studies fail to show this statistical association between agricultural work and ALS.[32,34] A recent systemic literature review by Sutedja and colleagues[88] also showed a significantly increased risk estimate for insecticides, fertilizers, other agricultural chemicals, and farm-related occupations. Moreover, these findings corroborate the hypothesis that exposure to pesticides and consequent mitochondrial dysfunction plays a role in the pathogenesis of ALS and other neurodegenerative disorders. On the contrary, Weisskopf and colleagues[89] performed a prospective study that did not find an association between ALS mortality and self-reported exposure to pesticides/herbicides, although there was some indication that those reporting 4 or more years of such exposure may be at increased risk. Therefore, these data do not clearly delineate whether this risk relates to chemical exposures, physical exertion, infections, or some other factor.

Solvents

In the study by Deapen and Henderson,[37] occupational exposures to toxins were similar for patients and controls except for plastics manufacturing. Their OR was 3.7, but with broad CIs. A subsequent study implicated solvents, but did not reach statistical significance. The Scottish Motor Neuron Disease Register case-control study published in 1993 did find a statistically significant increased risk (OR, 3.3; 95% CI, 1.3–10) of exposure to chemicals/solvents, but again with wide CIs.[35] Two other studies have failed to replicate these weak findings.[38,39] In their large prospective study, Weisskopf and colleagues[89] found evidence suggesting an increased risk of ALS with formaldehyde exposure, including a strong trend with increasing years of exposure. Because of the longitudinal design of the study, this finding is unlikely to be caused by bias, but it should nevertheless be interpreted cautiously and needs to be independently verified.[89] Thus, the role of solvent exposure to development of ALS seems small.

Cigarette Smoking

A myriad of toxins are associated with cigarette smoking. These toxins might play a role in causing or triggering ALS, possibly by inducing oxidative stress. To the contrary, smoking was previously believed to hold a potentially protective effect on the development of Parkinson disease and Alzheimer disease.[90] Early studies found no association of ALS with smoking.[32,38,91] In the late 1990s, 3 case-control studies obtained positive, although weak, associations for previous or current cigarette smoking and ALS.[47,92,93] Nelson and colleagues[93] found associations with ever smoking cigarettes (OR, 2.0; with a narrow 95% CI of 1.3, 3.2), current smoking (threefold risk), and significant trends for increased risk of ALS with duration of smoking and number of cigarette pack-years. Their study was a large case-control study with 161 incident cases and 321 matched controls. A prospective study based in New England assessed the relation between cigarette smoking and ALS mortality among the participants in the Cancer Prevention Study II and found conflicting results. Among 291 woman and 330 men who died of ALS between 1989 and 1998, the relative risk of death from ALS among current smokers compared with never smokers was 1.67 (95% CI, 1.24–2.24) for women and 0.69 (95% CI, 0.49, 0.99) for men. These diametrically opposite results suggest that cigarette smoking may increase the likelihood of ALS in women, but not men (and may even be protective). A more recent study of 364 patients and 392 controls shows that currently smoking cigarettes is an independent risk factor for sporadic ALS. In this study, both male and female current smokers showed an increased risk of ALS.[94] Thus, the data suggest a mild risk associated with smoking.

GULF WAR SERVICE

A decade after the end of the 1990 to 1991 Persian Gulf War, 2 studies observed an increased incidence of ALS in military personnel with deployment to the Persian Gulf region. Horner and colleagues[95] derived an increased relative risk (RR) for all deployed personnel (RR, 1.92; 95% CI, 1.29, 2.84), deployed active duty military (RR, 2.15; 95% CI, 1.38, 3.36), deployed Air Force members (RR, 2.68; 95% CI, 1.24, 5.78), and deployed Army troops (RR, 2.04; 95% CI, 1.10, 3.77). Subgroup analyses found that increased risks did not reach statistical significance for populations of deployed Marine, Army National Guard, or Navy personnel. Halsey[96] studied ALS in young Gulf War veterans (age >45 years). He reported that ALS incidence rates in young veterans exceeded that expected from age-specific United States population death rates.[96]

Early studies of Persian Gulf War veterans failed to find increased rates of illness. One found no excess of unexplained hospitalizations.[97] Deployed veterans had a slightly, but significantly, higher death rate after deployment, but most of this increased mortality was related to accidents and not disease.[98] A later review of hospitalization records looked specifically at systemic lupus erythematosus, fibromyalgia, and ALS.[99] That study concluded that Gulf War veterans were hospitalized slightly more often for fibromyalgia, but not for lupus. The data for ALS were inconclusive because of small numbers and wide CIs. In 2001, a case-control study drawing from Department of Veterans Affairs and the Social Security Administration databases found a nonsignificant deficit of deaths caused by ALS (RR, 0.59; 95% CI,0.21, 1.66).[100] The epidemiologic strengths of these studies suffer from their small numbers of ALS cases and several potential methodological issues, some of which are unavoidable. The most recent and comprehensive study compared death from brain tumors, ALS, multiple sclerosis and Parkinson disease in Gulf War veterans compared with veterans who did not serve in Gulf War I.[101] In the 13-year period from 1991 to 2004, and with more than 500,000 persons in each cohort, no association was found for ALS.

Thorough electrophysiologic evaluations of Gulf War veterans with neuromuscular symptoms have failed to discern objective measurable abnormalities in veterans from the United States[102] or the United Kingdom.[103] Cases of ALS were not found in these series. Several environmental factors have been purported to possibly initiate or cause ALS in military personnel deployed to the Persian Gulf: pesticides, chemical weapons, immunizations, medications, radiation exposure, physical exertion, trauma, genetic predisposition, or some unique interplay of these factors. Thus far, none have strong evidence supporting causation. An examination of archived records of hospitalizations in United States military facilities in the Kuwait theater of operations and European evacuation facilities showed no increase in the OR for exposure to smoke from oil well fires or possible nerve agent exposure.[104]

The possible role of toxins (which included nerve agent exposure, and so forth) in the Gulf War syndrome have been explored in more detail.[105] In late 2004, the Research Advisory Committee on Gulf War Veterans' Illnesses, a congressionally chartered panel of scientific experts and veterans, released its first major report on Gulf War illnesses. The report concluded that a substantial proportion of Gulf War veterans suffer from unexplained illnesses; these illnesses are not explained by stress or psychiatric illness in most cases; ill veterans exhibit an excess of ALS; research supports a probable link to neurotoxic exposures; treatments are urgently needed; and further research is imperative for military missions and homeland security.[106] In November 2008, the Research Advisory Committee on Gulf War Veterans' Illnesses published its second report. They again affirmed the existence of Gulf War syndrome as a distinct entity and a higher prevalence of ALS in Gulf War I veterans. The committee did note that there was the appearance of a time-limited disease outbreak in veterans in the decade following the Gulf War.[107] The highest risk was observed in 1996, and declined thereafter.[108]

Cox and colleagues[109] suggest that inhalation of β-N-methylamino-l-alanine (BMAA), and 2,4 diaminobutyric acid (DAB), and other cyanotoxins may be linked to the observed increase in ALS in military personnel deployed to the Gulf from 1990 to 1991. Their data indicate that biologic soil crusts, in this case dominated by cyanobacteria, cover significant portions of the flat desert areas. The dried crusts contain neurotoxic cyanobacterial toxins including BMAA and DAB. If dust containing cyanobacteria is inhaled, significant exposure to BMAA and other cyanotoxins may occur. They suggest that inhalation of BMAA, DAB, and other aerosolized cyanotoxins may constitute a significant risk factor for the development of ALS in this group.

The association of ALS with the Gulf War remains a lightning rod issue with evidence both in favor of, and not supportive of, an increased incidence of ALS in Gulf War veterans.

INFECTIONS

One prominent early theory concerning the cause of ALS was that of an underlying viral agent causing the disease directly, indirectly, or in a latent state. An early case-control study found a history of polio in 5 of 80 patients with ALS, and none of 78 controls.[32] However, large case-control studies failed to find any association between previous polio infection and ALS risk,[110] and a review of the epidemiologic literature came to the same determination. Detection of enterovirus nucleic acid sequences via polymerase chain reaction in cerebrospinal fluid[111] and neuronal cell bodies[112] of spinal cords of patients with ALS reignited interest in this mechanism of disease. However, other researchers have been unable to reproduce these findings.[113,114] Retroviral infection may cause motor neuron disease with either lower or both upper and lower motor neuron involvement, and this occurs in human T cell leukemic virus 1 (HTLV-1) infection[115] and also in human immunodeficiency virus disease.[116,117] Treatment of the underlying HIV infection can transiently or completely reverse the associated motor neuron disease.[116–118] A poliomyelitis like syndrome with an asymmetric lower motor neuronopathy may accompany West Nile virus infection, with or without meningoencephalitis.[119] Hepatitis C infection may also produce a pure motor axonal polyneuropathy without cryoglobulinemia that is at least somewhat responsive to therapy for the underlying viral infection.[120] Lower motor neuron involvement occasionally accompanies the prion disorders, Creutzfeldt-Jacob disease and Gerstmann-Sträussler-Scheinker disease.[121] With reports that Lyme disease rarely presents as a motor neuronopathy,[122] and that spirochetes have been cultured from cases with ALS,[123] bacterial infections have been postulated as potential causes of, or triggers for, ALS.[124] Approaching the issue of a bacterial cause from a treatment perspective, a trial of ceftriaxone therapy in ALS lacked efficacy.[125] The antibiotic minocycline had initially shown benefit in slowing ALS in mouse models, but this positive effect was not believed to be caused by the drug's antibacterial effects, but rather its neuroprotective actions.[126–128] A multicentre, randomized, placebo-controlled phase III trial by Gordon and colleagues[129] had 412 patients randomly assigned to receive placebo or minocycline in escalating doses of up to 400 mg/d MPW for 9 months. The primary outcome measure was the difference in rate of change in the revised ALS functional rating scale (ALSFRS-R). ALSFRS-R score deterioration was faster in the minocycline group than in the placebo group (-1.30 vs -1.04 units/mo; 95% CI for difference -0.44 to -0.08; $P = .005$). More investigation is required before a bacterial theory gains credulity. At this time, any relation between infections and the cause of ALS must be viewed as speculative and unsubstantiated.

NEOPLASMS

Patients with ALS may also develop cancer. An association between lymphoma and a lower motor neuron disorder has been reported. Some cases present signs of classic ALS with evidence of upper and lower motor neuron disease.[130] Patients with other cancers also manifest ALS-like symptoms.[131] Infrequently, patients who initially present with PLS and breast cancer eventually develop both upper and lower motor neuron dysfunction.[132] Motor neuron disease may also be a manifestation of a paraneoplastic syndrome. Anti-Hu antibodies[133] and anti-Yo antibodies[134] are associated with cases of motor neuron disease. These cases remain rare in the literature. Vigliani and colleagues[135] published a case-control study of patients with ALS with cancer using patients with ALS without cancer as controls. In their study, patients with ALS with and without cancer did not significantly differ clinically. Patients with

ALS with cancer die of motor neuron disease irrespective of cancer progression. Treatment with antitumor therapy does not influence the course of their ALS.

Exceptional cases of a lower motor neuron disorder may be related to underlying cancers; however, the coexistence of ALS and cancer in most cases is random.

ELECTRICAL SHOCK AND ELECTROMAGNETIC FIELDS

Instances of myeloradiculopathy as a delayed neurologic consequence of electrical injuries spurred conjecture as to the association of electrical trauma and ALS.[136] Two case-control studies from the 1980s described a greater association of electrical injury in patients with ALS compared with controls.[37,137] A nationwide Danish mortality study conducted a comparison of all men employed in utility companies from 1900 to 1993 and compared them with national death rates for different causes. This utility worker study found a twofold increase in mortality from ALS and a tenfold increase in deaths from electrical accidents. They postulate that the increased exposure to electrical shocks and electromagnetic fields (EMFs) may be causally associated with the excess mortality from ALS.[138] The Scottish Motor Neuron Disease Register study found no such association between ALS and electrical injury in Scotland.[35]

The hypothesis is that electrical injuries may simply parallel EMF exposure, thus serving as a surrogate marker. Davanipour and colleagues[139] conducted a case-control study investigating lifetime occupational exposure to EMFs in 28 patients with ALS. The ORs for total occupational exposure and average occupational exposure to EMFs in patients with at least 20 years of work experience were 7.5 (95% CI, 1.4, 38.1) and 5.5 (95% CI, 1.3, 22.5), respectively. The broad CIs weaken the strength of this association in this small population. When the comparison was extended to all patients with ALS regardless of total work experience, the ORs did not meet statistical significance. Savitz and colleagues[140,141] performed a mortality study in United States utility workers and a case-control study of the neurodegenerative disorders, Parkinson disease, Alzheimer disease, and ALS in these same workers. Both studies found weak associations between ALS and extent of EMF exposure. A Scandinavian case-referent study found ALS to be associated with a history of electrical occupation (OR, 2.30; 95% CI, 1.29, 4.09) but not with EMF exposure as estimated by a job-exposure matrix.[142] Contradictory results were obtained in 2 publications using predominantly the same Swedish study populations. Håkansson and colleagues[143] reported a relative risk of 2.2 (95% CI, 1.0, 4.7) for EMF exposure and ALS, whereas Feychting and colleagues[144] failed to discover any such association. Plausible biologic mechanisms linking EMFs to the onset of ALS remain poorly understood. If EMFs do increase the risk of ALS, that risk seems small.

PHYSICAL FACTORS

Physical exertion, participation in athletics, bodily trauma, bone fractures, and surgeries have all been posited to be antecedent events more common in patients with ALS than in controls. Famous athletes have developed ALS, and their popularity may highlight this association in peoples' minds despite no true association or causation. However, this prominence of athletes in a culture's collective mind has led to use of the term Lou Gehrig's disease for ALS in the United States. Possible mechanism(s) underlying this relationship include increased exposure to ambient toxins, greater contact of neural tissues with immune surveillance systems, augmented absorption or bodily distribution of toxins, and neuronal fatigue and stress. Numerous studies support this general hypothesis,[31,33,35,37,38,47,88,91,145] whereas others were not able to substantiate the association.[34,109,146,147] Physical exertion and trauma remain one mechanism possibly underlying risk of ALS in Gulf War veterans. An intriguing development is the clustering of ALS in Italian soccer players. From 1960 to 1997, approximately 24,000 men played professional soccer, of whom 8 already died of ALS.[148] The true number of players suffering or dying from ALS is believed to be greater than 30.[149] The expected number of cases in the Italian general population in the age group of the soccer players would be less than 1 case. Disease onset in these athletes is usually in their 40s. The mechanism of disease onset in these soccer players is not yet known. They suffer more head trauma and bone fractures and are more physically active than the general population. The literature provides some evidence for the involvement of head injury in patients with ALS.[91] Other studies do not support trauma as a causal factor, but point toward physical exertion.[150] It is not clear whether these athletes use performance enhancing drugs at a greater frequency than the general population, but this would be a safe assumption. Therefore, a toxic cause should also be considered. Another hypothesis posits the existence of some genetic factor initially providing athletic excellence only to culminate in premature neuronal degeneration. No such gene is yet known.

Inclusions positive for TDP-43 are seen in cases of ALS, whereas tau is present in frontotemporal dementia. A recent study found that 3 of 12 patients with chronic traumatic encephalopathy (CTE) also had ALS. The finding of TDP-43 and tau in neuronal inclusions in both spinal cord and brain of these patients with ALS was interpreted to suggest trauma as a cause of the motor neuron disease.[151] Issues of ascertainment bias led to questions about simple coincident occurrence of 2 diseases and doubt as to causality. In a large case-control series, Turner and colleagues[152] noted an increased likelihood of head or extremity trauma requiring hospitalization in patients with ALS; however, this increase in trauma was only during the year before diagnosis. Their interpretation of these data was that the trauma was most likely to be a consequence of incipient ALS, not the cause of the ALS.

At the current time, the association between physical exertion and trauma and the development of ALS remains captivating, but without powerful epidemiologic support or a proven pathogenic mechanism.

DIET

Ingestion of certain foods, toxins associated with foods, or toxins within foods might predispose to development of ALS. In Texas, Felmus and colleagues[31] found that consumption of large quantities of milk was associated with patients with ALS.[32] As a prominent source of calcium, milk might affect absorption or body stores of heavy metals and could alter parathyroid function. Parathyroid disease causes weakness, exercise intolerance, and muscle atrophy, but is now known not to be associated with ALS. Two more case-control studies failed to find an association with milk ingestion or with any particular food.[33,146] A large case-control study from Washington State in the United States found that high amounts of dietary fat intake correlated with ALS (OR, 2.7; 95% CI, 0.9, 8.0), whereas high dietary fiber intake appeared protective (OR, 0.3; 95% CI, 0.1, 0.7).[153] High glutamate intake was also linked with an increased risk of ALS (OR, 3.2; 95% CI, 1.2, 8.0). Consumption of dietary or supplemental antioxidant vitamins did not decrease this hazard. These glutamate findings follow in step with the glutamate excitotoxicity theory of ALS, whereas the data on fats and fiber fit well with a model related to toxin ingestion.

Lathyrism is a neurologic disorder with predominant upper motor neuron dysfunction associated with the use of the chickling pea (*Lathyrus sativa*) in foodstuffs. A drought-resistant crop, the chickling pea contains abundant quantities of b-N-oxalyl-l-a,b-diaminopropionic acid (b-ODAP), a glutamate analogue, which is believed to cause neuronal damage via excitation of the AMPA-activated receptors. Another neurologic disorder, konzo, is a tropical myelopathy presenting with abrupt onset of spastic paraplegia.[154] Consumption of flour from insufficiently processed cassava leads to excessive dietary cyanide exposure and resultant disease. In addition, an atypical parkinsonism in the French West Indies is associated with consumption of herbal teas and fruits from the Annonaceae family that contain neurotoxic benzyltetrahydroisoquinoline alkaloids.[155] Four of 30 patients with this atypical parkinsonism had associated motor neuron disease. The neuronal toxicity of benzyltetrahydroisoquinolines is believed to be mediated either through glutamate toxicity or free radical formation. Recently, in a large prospective study, Morozova and colleagues[156] did not find convincing evidence that food items are related to ALS mortality. Although the results suggested a possible protective effect of high chicken consumption, studies in other populations are needed to determine whether this association is reproducible.

WESTERN PACIFIC ALS

Three foci in the western Pacific, Guam, the Kii Peninsula of Japan, and western New Guinea, were determined to have markedly increased rates of ALS in the middle of the last century.[157] In the 1940s and 1950s, the annual incidence rates for the Chamorro natives on the island of Guam were 50 per 100,000, with incidence rates in certain municipalities or districts as high as 250 per 100,000.[158] These Guamanian ALS incidence rates were as much as 100-fold increased compared with age-adjusted worldwide incidence rates. Prevalence rates reached nearly 1 in 600 Guamanian Chamorros of all ages and almost 1 in 100 for persons in their 40s and 50s. Native Chamorros, who called their ALS syndrome by the name of lytico, also were aware of a concomitant disease running in their populations, a PDC with the Chamorran name of bodig. These 2 diseases may occur concurrently in the same patient or same family, leading to the term ALS-PDC. Although incidence rates for ALS in the western Pacific have substantially decreased with time, distinct foci continue to exceed worldwide values.[159] Postmortem pathologic specimens of patients with ALS and PDC reveal pyknosis and loss of anterior horn cells in the spinal cord and neurofibrillary degeneration in the cortex.[160]

Investigators proposed 3 main theories explaining the high incidence of western Pacific ALS: a genetic underpinning in this isolated island population caused by familial aggregation of cases of both ALS and PDC[161]; dietary consumption of a plant neurotoxin from the cycad plant in the form of cycad flour[162,163]; or exposure to drinking water and agricultural soil low in calcium and high in aluminum.[63] Although western Pacific ALS arose 7 to 28 times more frequently in siblings of patients with ALS than in the Chamorro population as a whole, ALS also occurred more often in spousal pairs.[164,165] This risk of ALS in susceptible sibships was still significantly lower than would be expected by a monogenic mendelian model. Polygenic inheritance, without an environmental trigger, was also unlikely. Thus, the increased ALS incidence in family members related either by blood or marriage fits better with a shared environmental exposure than with a purely genetic cause. Even with substantial influx of other races onto the island of Guam, with intermixing of gene pools in the past 50 years, much more generational time would have had to pass to explain the marked decline in incidence.[166] Evaluation of the case registry on Guam by Zhang and colleagues[164] determined that the cycad neurotoxin hypothesis better conformed with the data than the low-calcium, high-aluminum hypothesis.

In 1963, Whiting[167] suggested that ALS on Guam might be related to ingestion of the seed of the false sago palm (*Cycas circinalis*). Much attention was initially given to cycasin, a potent hepatotoxic and carcinogenic component of the cycad seed. Spencer and colleagues[162] subsequently proposed that BMAA may be the offending agent in cycad seeds. This group orally administered BMAA to cynomolgus monkeys, inducing neurologic dysfunction with upper and lower motor neuron involvement. These monkeys also developed chromatolytic and degenerative changes of motor neurons in the cerebral cortex and spinal cord.[163] The main exposure of the native Chamorro people to these toxins was through consumption of flour made from the cycad seeds. The Chamorro people subjected the cycad seeds for flour to multiple washings for detoxification, because they knew these seeds to be acutely toxic. Processed cycad flour contains very little BMAA.[168] Therefore humans would need to eat massive quantities of flour-based foods on a daily basis. With this information, cycad flour fell out of favor as a potential source for a neurotoxin in Guamanian ALS.

The exact substance in cycad seeds exerting the neurotoxic effect is still being debated.[169] However, the mechanism by which the Chamorro people were exposed to these neurotoxins may now be resolved. ALS-PDC seems to be the product of biomagnification of neurotoxins up through the food chain.[170] Guamanian flying foxes (*Pteropus mariannus mariannus*) consume large quantities of the BMAA-laden sarcotesta of cycad seeds. Museum specimens of Guamanian flying foxes contain high levels of BMAA, levels 1000 times more concentrated than in cycad seed flour.[171] The Chamorro people traditionally feasted on flying foxes, and consumption of a single flying fox may have resulted in a dose of BMAA equivalent to 174 to 1014 kg of processed cycad flour. Flying foxes may therefore be the entry route for massive quantities of a neurotoxin leading to the subsequent development of ALS-PDC. Cox and colleagues[172] further detailed this biomagnification by documenting the following progressive concentrating effect on BMAA upward through the food chain: (1) freeliving cyanobacteria produce 0.3 µg/g BMAA; (2) cyanobacteria living as symbionts in cycad roots produce 2 to 37 µg/g BMAA; (3) cycad seeds contain mean levels of 1161 µg/g BMAA in their fleshy outer seed layer; (4) flying fox tissues accumulate mean levels of 3556 µg/g BMAA. Frontal cortex from 6 Chamorro patients who died of ALS-PDC contained mean BMAA levels of 6 µg/g. BMAA was also extracted from the frontal cortices of 2 Canadian patients with Alzheimer disease at autopsy with mean levels of 6.6 µg/g. BMAA was not detected in frontal cortex from postmortem evaluation of 13 Canadian patients without neurodegenerative diseases. BMAA exists in both free and bound forms in bacterial, plant, animal, and human tissues. Protein-bound BMAA levels may be 1 to 2 orders of magnitude higher than free BMAA levels. Protein-bound BMAA levels in brain tissues from Guamanian patients with ALS-PDC ranged from 60-fold to 130-fold higher than free levels.[173] BMAA bound to protein may function as an endogenous neurotoxic reservoir, and this reservoir may even be neuroprotective. Large doses of neurotoxin might acutely be absorbed and sequestered in protein-bound form, only to be slowly discharged into the surrounding brain milieu.

Biomagnification of neurotoxins seems a strong candidate to explain ALS-PDC of Guam. Further investigations into biomagnification of other neurotoxins in ALS and other neurodegenerative disorders might elucidate a novel mechanism for neural degeneration.

EDUCATION/SOCIOECONOMIC STATUS

Levels of education or socioeconomic status have only infrequently been studied as risk factors for ALS. Two case-control studies showed inconsistent findings.[35,38]

A large population-based study showed a lack of association between social class of patients with ALS and controls.[35] An older case-control study performed between 1964 and 1982 showed a low level of education to be associated with an increased risk of ALS.[38] Other epidemiologic studies have suggested both an increased risk of ALS with higher levels of education[174] and a lack of association of level of education with ALS.[175] However, these studies did not adjust for smoking and so a higher prevalence of smoking among lower socioeconomic groups may provide the explanation for these inconsistent findings.[176]

SUMMARY

Environmental exposures in sporadic ALS remain mostly associations without causation. More than 20 genetic loci are known to be responsible for cases of familial motor neuron disease. Research into sporadic ALS suggests that numerous factors may be contributory in the disease process, but a singular cause and unifying pathogenesis remain elusive. A multitude of genetic, toxic, autoimmune, infectious, and systemic processes may be at play in ALS, similar to muscle diseases, neuromuscular junction disorders, and polyneuropathies.

REFERENCES

1. Rowland LP, Shneider NA. Amyotrophic lateral sclerosis. N Engl J Med 2001; 344:1688–700.
2. Lomen-Hoerth C, Murphy J, Langmore S, et al. Are amyotrophic lateral sclerosis patients cognitively normal? Neurology 2003;60:1094–7.
3. Leigh PN, Ray-Chaudhury K. Motor neuron disease. J Neurol Neurosurg Psychiatry 1994;57:886–96.
4. Govoni V, Granieri E, Capone J, et al. Incidence of amyotrophic lateral sclerosis in the local health district of Ferrara, Italy, 1964-1998. Neuroepidemiology 2003; 22:229–34.
5. Chancellor AM, Warlow CP. Adult onset motor neuron disease: worldwide mortality, incidence and distribution since 1950. J Neurol Neurosurg Psychiatry 1992;55:1106–15.
6. Brooks BR. El Escorial World Federation of Neurology criteria for the diagnosis of amyotrophic lateral sclerosis. J Neurol Sci 1994;124(Suppl):96–107.
7. Brooks BR, Miller RG, Swash M, et al. World Federation of Neurology Research Group on Motor Neuron Diseases. El Escorial revisited: revised criteria for the diagnosis of amyotrophic lateral sclerosis. Amyotroph Lateral Scler Other Motor Neuron Disord 2000;1:293–9.
8. de Carvalho M, Dengler M, Eisen A, et al. Electrodiagnostic criteria for diagnosis of ALS. Clin Neurophysiol 2008;119:497–503.
9. Okita T, Nodura H, Shibuta Y, et al. Can Awaji ALS criteria provide earlier diagnosis than the revised El Escorial criteria? J Neurol Sci 2011;302:29–32.
10. Triggs WJ, Menkes D, Onorato J, et al. Transcranial magnetic stimulation identifies upper motor neuron involvement in motor neuron disease. Neurology 1999; 53:605–11.
11. Sach M, Winkler G, Glauche V, et al. Diffusion tensor MRI of early upper motor neuron involvement in amyotrophic lateral sclerosis. Brain 2004;127:340–50.
12. Olney RK, Yuen EC, Engstrom JW. Statistical motor unit number estimation: reproducibility and sources of error in patients with amyotrophic lateral sclerosis. Muscle Nerve 2000;23:193–7.
13. Ross MA. Acquired motor neuron disorders. Neurol Clin 1997;3:481–500.

14. Bensimon G, Lacomblez L, Meinenger V. A controlled trial of riluzole in amyotrophic lateral sclerosis. N Engl J Med 1994;330:585–91.
15. Siddique T, Pericak-Vance MA, Brooks BR, et al. Linkage analysis in familial amyotrophic lateral sclerosis. Neurology 1989;39:919–25.
16. Rosen DR, Siddique T, Patterson D, et al. Mutations in copper/zinc superoxide dismutase gene are associated with familial amyotrophic lateral sclerosis. Nature 1993;362:59–62.
17. Siddique T, Lalani I. Genetic aspects of amyotrophic lateral sclerosis. In: Pourmand R, Harati Y, editors. Neuromuscular disorders, vol. 88. Philadelphia: Williams & Wilkins; 2002.
18. Majoor-Krakauer D, Willems PJ, Hofman A. Genetic epidemiology of amyotrophic lateral sclerosis. Clin Genet 2003;63:83–101.
19. Neuromuscular Disease Center Website. Hereditary Motor Syndromes Page. St Louis (MO): Washington University. Available at: http://www.neuro.wustl.edu/neuromuscular/synmot.html#Hereditaryals. Accessed June 12, 2011.
20. Al-Chalabi A, Anderson PM, Chioza B, et al. Recessive amyotrophic lateral sclerosis families with the D90A SOD1 mutation share a common founder: evidence for a linked protective factor. Hum Mol Genet 1998;7:2045–50.
21. Ratovitski T, Corson LB, Strain J, et al. Variation in the biochemical/biophysical properties of mutant superoxide dismutase 1 enzymes and the rate of disease progression in familial amyotrophic lateral sclerosis kindreds. Hum Mol Genet 1999;8:1451–60.
22. Reaume AG, Elliott JL, Hoffman EK, et al. Motor neurons in Cu/Zn superoxide dismutase-deficient mice develop normally but exhibit enhanced cell death after axonal injury. Nat Genet 1996;13:43–7.
23. Jones CT, Swingler RJ, Simpson SA, et al. Superoxide dismutase mutations in an unselected cohort of Scottish amyotrophic lateral sclerosis patients. J Med Genet 1995;32:290–2.
24. Jackson M, Al-Chalabi A, Enayat ZE, et al. Copper/zinc superoxide dismutase 1 and sporadic amyotrophic lateral sclerosis: analysis of 155 cases and identification of a novel insertion mutation. Ann Neurol 1997;42:803–7.
25. Puls I, Jonnakuty C, LaMonte BH, et al. Mutant dynactin in motor neuron disease. Nat Genet 2003;33:455–6.
26. Callaghan B, Feldman D, Gruis K, et al. The association of exposure to lead, mercury, and selenium and the development of amyotrophic lateral sclerosis and the epigenetic implications. Neurodegener Dis 2011;8:1–8.
27. Wilson SA. The amyotrophy of chronic lead poisoning – amyotrophic lateral sclerosis of toxic origin. Rev Neurol Psychiatry 1907;5:441–55.
28. Mishra D, Agrawal A, Gupta VK. Distal spinal muscular atrophy of upper limb (Hirayama disease) associated with high serum lead levels. Indian Pediatr 2003;40:780–3.
29. Livesley B, Sissons CE. Chronic lead intoxication mimicking motor neurone disease. BMJ 1968;4:387–8.
30. Boothby JA, DeJesus PV, Rowland LP. Reversible forms of motor neuron disease: lead "neuritis". Arch Neurol 1974;31:18–23.
31. Felmus MT, Patten BM, Swanke L. Antecedent events in amyotrophic lateral sclerosis. Neurology 1976;26:167–72.
32. Pierce-Ruhland R, Patten BM. Repeat study of antecedent events in motor neuron disease. Ann Clin Res 1981;13:102–7.
33. Roelofs-Iverson RA, Mulder DW, Elveback LR, et al. ALS and heavy metals: a pilot case-control study. Neurology 1984;34:393–5.

34. Armon C, Kurland LT, Daube JR, et al. Epidemiologic correlates of sporadic amyotrophic lateral sclerosis. Neurology 1991;41:1077–84.
35. Chancellor AM, Slattery JM, Fraser H, et al. Risk factors for motor neuron disease: a case-control study based on patients from the Scottish Motor Neuron Disease Register. J Neurol Neurosurg Psychiatry 1993;56:1200–6.
36. Fang F, Kwee LC, Allen KD, et al. Association between blood lead and the risk of amyotrophic lateral sclerosis. Am J Epidemiol 2010;171:1126–33.
37. Deapen DM, Henderson BE. A case-control study of amyotrophic lateral sclerosis. Am J Epidemiol 1986;123:790–9.
38. Granieri E, Carreras M, Tola R, et al. Motor neuron disease in the province of Ferrara, Italy, in 1964-1982. Neurology 1988;38:1604–8.
39. McGuire V, Longstreth WT, Nelson LM, et al. Occupational exposures and amyotrophic lateral sclerosis: a population-based case-control study. Am J Epidemiol 1997;145:1076–88.
40. Conradi S, Ronnevi LO, Vesterberg O. Abnormal tissue distribution of lead in amyotrophic lateral sclerosis. J Neurol Sci 1976;29:259–65.
41. Conradi S, Ronnevi LO, Vesterberg O. Abnormal distribution of lead in amyotrophic lateral sclerosis: reestimation of lead in the cerebrospinal fluid. J Neurol Sci 1980;48:413–8.
42. Conradi S, Ronnevi LO, Vesterberg O. Increased plasma levels of lead in patients with amyotrophic lateral sclerosis compared with control subjects as determined by flameless atomic absorption spectrophotometry. J Neurol Neurosurg Psychiatry 1978;41:389–93.
43. Petkau A, Sawatzky A, Hillier CR, et al. Lead content of neuromuscular tissue in amyotrophic lateral sclerosis: case report and other considerations. Br J Ind Med 1974;31:275–87.
44. Conradi S, Ronnevi LO, Vesterberg O. Lead concentration in skeletal muscle in amyotrophic lateral sclerosis patients and control subjects. J Neurol Neurosurg Psychiatry 1978;41:1001–4.
45. Kurlander HM, Patten BM. Metals in spinal cord tissue of patients dying of motor neuron disease. Ann Neurol 1979;6:21–4.
46. Mandybur TI, Cooper GP. Increased spinal cord lead content in amyotrophic lateral sclerosis – possibly a secondary phenomenon. Med Hypotheses 1979;5:1313–5.
47. Vinceti M, Guidetti D, Bergomi M, et al. Lead, cadmium, and selenium in the blood of patients with sporadic amyotrophic lateral sclerosis. Ital J Neurol Sci 1997;18:87–92.
48. Pamphlett R, McQuilty R, Zarkos K. Blood levels of toxic and essential metals in motor neuron disease. Neurotoxicology 2001;22:401–10.
49. Bergomi M, Vinceti M, Nacci G, et al. Environmental exposure to trace elements and risk of amyotrophic lateral sclerosis: a population-based case-control study. Environ Res 2002;89:116–23.
50. Currier RD, Haerer AF. Amyotrophic lateral sclerosis and metal toxins. Arch Environ Health 1968;17:712–9.
51. House AO, Abbott RJ, Davidson DL, et al. Response to penicillamine of lead concentrations in CSF and blood of patients with motor neurone disease. Br Med J 1978;2:1684.
52. Conradi S, Ronnevi LO, Nise G, et al. Long-time penicillamine treatment in amyotrophic lateral sclerosis with parallel determination of lead in blood, plasma and urine. Acta Neurol Scand 1982;65:203–11.

53. Brown IA. Chronic mercurialism. A cause of the clinical syndrome of amyotrophic lateral sclerosis. AMA Arch Neurol Psychiatry 1954;72:674–81.
54. Kantarjian AD. A syndrome clinically resembling amyotrophic lateral sclerosis following chronic mercurialism. Neurology 1961;11:639–44.
55. Barber TE. Inorganic mercury intoxication reminiscent of amyotrophic lateral sclerosis. J Occup Med 1978;20:667–9.
56. Adams CA, Ziegler DK, Lin JT. Mercury intoxication simulating amyotrophic lateral sclerosis. JAMA 1983;250:642–3.
57. Schwarz S, Husstedt IW, Bertram HP, et al. Amyotrophic lateral sclerosis after accidental injection of mercury. J Neurol Neurosurg Psychiatry 1996;60:698.
58. Gresham LS, Molgaard CA, Golbeck AL, et al. Amyotrophic lateral sclerosis and occupational heavy metal exposure: a case control study. Neuroepidemiology 1986;5:29–38.
59. Pamphlett R, Waley P. Mercury in human spinal motor neurons. Acta Neuropathol 1998;96:515–9.
60. Yase Y. The pathogenesis of amyotrophic lateral sclerosis. Lancet 1972;2(7772): 292–6.
61. Garruto RM, Yanagihara R, Gajdusek DC, et al. Concentration of heavy metals and essential minerals in garden soil and drinking water in the Western Pacific. In: Chen KM, Yase Y, editors. Amyotrophic lateral sclerosis in Asia and Oceania. Taipei (Taiwan): Shyan-Fu Chou: National Taiwan University; 1984. p. 265–329.
62. Perl DP, Gajdusek DC, Garruto RM, et al. Intraneuronal aluminum accumulation in amyotrophic lateral sclerosis and parkinsonism-dementia of Guam. Science 1982;217:1053–5.
63. Garruto RM, Shankar SK, Yanagihara R, et al. Low-calcium, high-aluminum diet-induced motor neuron pathology in cynomolgus monkeys. Acta Neuropathol 1989;78:210–9.
64. Strong MJ, Garruto RM. Chronic aluminum-induced motor neuron degeneration: clinical, neuropathological and molecular biological aspects. Can J Neurol Sci 1991;18(Suppl 3):428–31.
65. Wakayama I, Nerurkar VR, Strong MJ, et al. Comparative study of chronic aluminum-induced neurofilamentous aggregates with intracytoplasmic inclusions of amyotrophic lateral sclerosis. Acta Neuropathol 1996;92:545–54.
66. Tanridag T, Coskun T, Hürdag C, et al. Motor neuron degeneration due to aluminum deposition in the spinal cord: a light microscopical study. Acta Histochem 1999;101:193–201.
67. Kihira T, Yoshida S, Yase Y, et al. Chronic low-Ca/Mg high-Al diet induces neuronal loss. Neuropathology 2002;22:152–60.
68. Kihira T, Yoshida S, Kondo T, et al. ALS-like skin changes in mice on a chronic low-Ca/Mg high-Al diet. J Neurol Sci 2004;219:7–14.
69. Kilness AW, Hochberg FH. Amyotrophic lateral sclerosis in a high selenium environment. JAMA 1976;237:2843–4.
70. Nagata H, Miyata S, Nakamura S, et al. Heavy metal concentrations in blood cells in patients with amyotrophic lateral sclerosis. J Neurol Sci 1985;67:173–8.
71. Mitchell JD, East BW, Harris IA, et al. Manganese, selenium and other trace elements in spinal cord, liver and bone in motor neurone disease. Eur Neurol 1991;31:7–11.
72. Vinceti M, Guidetti D, Pinotti M, et al. Amyotrophic lateral sclerosis after long-term exposure to drinking water with high selenium content. Epidemiology 1996;7:529–32.

73. Cotzias GC, Horiuchi K, Fuenzalida S, et al. Chronic manganese poisoning: clearance of tissue manganese concentrations with persistence of the neurological picture. Neurology 1968;18:376–82.

74. Parboosingh JS, Rouleau GA, Meninger V, et al. Absence of mutations in the Mn superoxide dismutase or catalase genes in familial amyotrophic lateral sclerosis. Neuromuscul Disord 1995;5:7–10.

75. Perry G, Sayre LM, Atwood CS, et al. The role of iron and copper in the aetiology of neurodegenerative disorders: therapeutic implications. CNS Drugs 2002;16: 339–52.

76. Chad D, Mitsumoto H, Adelman LS, et al. Conjugal motor neurone disease. Neurology 1982;32:306–7.

77. Camu W, Cadilhac J, Billiard M. Conjugal amyotrophic lateral sclerosis: a report on two couples from southern France. Neurology 1994;44:547–8.

78. Sienko DG, Davis JP, Taylor JA, et al. Amyotrophic lateral sclerosis: a case control study following detection of a cluster in a small Wisconsin community. Arch Neurol 1990;47:38–41.

79. Armon C, Daube JR, O'Brien PC, et al. When is an apparent excess of neurologic cases epidemiologically significant? Neurology 1991;41:1713–8.

80. Proctor SP, Feldman RG, Wolf PA, et al. A perceived cluster of amyotrophic lateral sclerosis in a Massachusetts community. Neuroepidemiology 1992;1: 277–81.

81. Mitchell JD, Gatrell AC, Al-Hamad A, et al. Geographical epidemiology of residence of patients with motor neuron disease in Lancashire and South Cumbria. J Neurol Neurosurg Psychiatry 1998;65:842–7.

82. Hyser CL, Kissel JT, Mendell JR. Three cases of amyotrophic lateral sclerosis in a common occupational environment. J Neurol 1987;234:443–4.

83. Mundt DJ, Dell LD, Luippold RS, et al. Cause-specific mortality among Kelly Air Force Base civilian employees, 1981-2001. J Occup Environ Med 2002;44: 989–96.

84. Ceroni M, Malasina A, Poloni TE, et al. Clustering of ALS patients in central Italy due to the occurrence of the L84F SOD1 gene mutation. Neurology 1999;53: 1064–71.

85. Rosati G, Pinna L, Granieri E, et al. Studies on epidemiological, clinical and etiological aspects of ALS disease in Sardinia, Southern Italy. Acta Neurol Scand 1977;55:231–44.

86. Giagheddu M, Puggioni G, Masala C, et al. Epidemiologic study of amyotrophic lateral sclerosis in Sardinia, Italy. Acta Neurol Scand 1983;68:394–404.

87. Chiò A, Meineri P, Tribolo A, et al. Risk factors in motor neuron disease: a case-control study. Neuroepidemiology 1991;10:174–84.

88. Sutedja NA, Veldink JH, Fischer K, et al. Exposure to chemicals and metals and risk of amyotrophic lateral sclerosis: a systematic review. Amyotroph Lateral Scler 2009;10:302–9.

89. Weisskopf MG, Morozova N, O'Reilly EJ, et al. Prospective study of chemical exposures and amyotrophic lateral sclerosis. J Neurol Neurosurg Psychiatry 2009;80:558–61.

90. Morens DM, Gradinetti A, Reed D, et al. Cigarette smoking and protection from Parkinson's disease: false association or etiologic clue. Neurology 1995;45:1041–51.

91. Kondo K, Tsubaki T. Case-control studies of motor neuron disease: association with mechanical injuries. Arch Neurol 1981;38:220–6.

92. Kamel F, Umbach DM, Munsat TL, et al. Association of cigarette smoking with amyotrophic lateral sclerosis. Neuroepidemiology 1999;18:194–202.

93. Nelson LM, McGuire V, Longstreth WT, et al. Population-based case-control study of amyotrophic lateral sclerosis in western Washington State. I. Cigarette smoking and alcohol consumption. Am J Epidemiol 2000;151:156–63.

94. Sutedja NA, Veldink JH, Fischer K, et al. Lifetime occupation, education, smoking, and risk of ALS. Neurology 2007;69:1508–14.

95. Horner RD, Kamins KG, Feussner JR, et al. Occurrence of amyotrophic lateral sclerosis among Gulf War veterans. Neurology 2003;61:742–9.

96. Halsey RW. Excess incidence of ALS in young Gulf War veterans. Neurology 2003;61:750–6.

97. Gray GC, Coate BD, Anderson CM, et al. The postwar hospitalization experience of U.S. veterans of the Persian Gulf War. N Engl J Med 1996;335:1505–13.

98. Kang HK, Bullman TA. Mortality among U.S. veterans of the Persian Gulf War. N Engl J Med 1996;335:1498–504.

99. Smith TC, Gray GC, Knoke JD. Is systemic lupus erythematosus, amyotrophic lateral sclerosis, or fibromyalgia associated with Persian Gulf War service? An examination of Department of Defense hospitalization data. Am J Epidemiol 2000;151:1053–9.

100. Kang HK, Bullman TA. Mortality among US veterans of the Persian Gulf War: 7-year follow up. Am J Epidemiol 2001;154:399–405.

101. Barth SK, Kang HK, Bullman TA, et al. Neurological mortality among U.S. veterans of the Gulf War: 13-year follow-up. Am J Ind Med 2009;52:663–70.

102. Amato AA, McVey A, Cha C, et al. Evaluation of neuromuscular symptoms in veterans of the Persian Gulf War. Neurology 1997;48:4–12.

103. Sharief MK, Priddin J, Delamont RS, et al. Neurophysiologic analysis of neuromuscular symptoms in UK Gulf War veterans. Neurology 2002;59:1518–25.

104. Smith TC, Corbeil TE, Ryan MA, et al. In-theater hospitalizations of US and allied personnel during the 1991 Gulf War. Am J Epidemiol 2004;159:1064–76.

105. Gronseth G. Gulf War Syndrome: a toxic exposure? A systematic review. Neurol Clin 2005;23:523–40.

106. Research Advisory Committee on Gulf War Veterans' Illnesses. Media release. Washington, DC: November 15, 2004.

107. Research Advisory Committee on Gulf War Veterans' Illnesses. Gulf war illness and the health of Gulf War veterans: scientific findings and recommendations. Washington, DC: US Government Printing Office; 2008.

108. Horner RD, Grambow SC, Coffman CJ, et al. Amyotrophic lateral sclerosis among 1991 Gulf War veterans: evidence for a time-limited outbreak. Neuroepidemiology 2008;31:28–32.

109. Cox PA, Richer R, Metcalf JS. Cyanobacteria and BMAA exposure from desert dust: a possible link to sporadic ALS among Gulf War veterans. Amyotroph Lateral Scler 2009;2:109–17.

110. Morikawa F, Okumura H, Tashiro K, et al. Motor neuron disease and past poliomyelitis. Geographic study in Hokaido, the northern-most island of Japan. J Neurol 1993;240:13–6.

111. Leparc-Goffart I, Julien J, Fuchs F, et al. Evidence for the presence of poliovirus genomic sequences in the CSF of patients with post-polio syndrome. J Clin Microbiol 1996;34:2023–36.

112. Berger MM, Kopp N, Vital C, et al. Detection and cellular localization of enterovirus RNA sequences in spinal cord of patients with ALS. Neurology 2000;54:20–5.

113. Swanson NR, Fox SA, Mastaglia FL. Search for persistent infection with poliovirus or other enteroviruses in amyotrophic lateral sclerosis-motor neuron disease. Neuromuscl Disord 1995;5:457–65.

114. Muir P, Nicholson F, Spencer GT, et al. Enterovirus infection of the central nervous system of humans: lack of an association with chronic neurological disease. J Gen Virol 1996;77:1469–76.

115. Roman GC. Neuroepidemiology of amyotrophic lateral sclerosis: clues to aetiology and pathogenesis. J Neurol Neurosurg Psychiatry 1996;61:131–7.

116. Moulignier A, Moulonguet A, Pialoux G, et al. Reversible ALS-like disorder in HIV infection. Neurology 2001;57:995–1001.

117. MacGowan DJ, Scelsa SN, Waldron M. An ALS-like syndrome with new HIV infection and complete response to antiretroviral therapy. Neurology 2001;57:1094–7.

118. Calza L, Manfredi R, Freo E, et al. Transient reversal of HIV-associated motor neuron disease following the introduction of highly active antiretroviral therapy. J Chemother 2004;16:98–101.

119. Leis AA, Stokic DS, Webb RM, et al. Clinical spectrum of muscle weakness in human West Nile virus infection. Muscle Nerve 2003;28:302–8.

120. Costa J, Resende C, de Carvalho M. Motor-axonal polyneuropathy with hepatitis C virus. Eur J Neurol 2003;10:183–5.

121. Worrall BB, Rowland LP, Chin SS, et al. Amyotrophy in prion diseases. Arch Neurol 2000;57:33–8.

122. Hemmer B, Glocker FX, Kaiser R, et al. Generalised motor neuron disease as an unusual manifestation of *Borrelia burgdorferi* infection. J Neurol Neurosurg Psychiatry 1997;63:257–8.

123. Mattman LH. Cell deficient forms: stealth pathogens. 3rd edition. Boca Raton (FL): CRC Press; 2001.

124. Koch AL. Cell wall-deficient (CWD) bacterial pathogens: could amyotrophic lateral sclerosis (ALS) be due to one? Crit Rev Microbiol 2003;29:215–21.

125. Robberecht W. Lack of improvement with ceftriaxone in motor neuron disease. Lancet 1992;340:1096–7.

126. Zhu S, Stavroskaya IG, Drozda M, et al. Minocycline inhibits cytochrome *c* release and delays progression of amyotrophic lateral sclerosis in mice. Nature 2002;417:74–8.

127. Van Den Bosch I, Tilkin P, Lemmens G, et al. Minocycline delays disease onset and mortality in a transgenic model of ALS. Neuroreport 2002;13:1067–70.

128. Kriz J, Nguyen M, Julien J. Minocycline slows disease progression in a mouse model of amyotrophic lateral sclerosis. Neurobiol Dis 2002;10:268.

129. Gordon PH, Moore DH, Miller RG. Efficacy of minocycline in patients with amyotrophic lateral sclerosis: a phase III randomised trial. Lancet Neurol 2007;6: 1045–53.

130. Younger DS, Rowland LP, Hays AP, et al. Lymphoma, motor neuron disease, and amyotrophic lateral sclerosis. Ann Neurol 1991;29:78–86.

131. Gordon PH, Rowland LP, Younger DS, et al. Lymphoproliferative disorders and motor neuron disease: an update. Neurology 1997;48:1671–8.

132. Forsythe PA, Dalmau J, Graus F, et al. Motor neuron syndromes in cancer patients. Ann Neurol 1997;41:722–30.

133. Verma A, Berger JR, Snodgrass S, et al. Motor neuron disease: a paraneoplastic process associated with anti-hu antibody and small-cell lung carcinoma. Ann Neurol 1996;40:112–6.

134. Khwaja S, Sripathi N, Ahmad BK, et al. Paraneoplastic motor neuron disease with type 1 Purkinje cell antibodies. Muscle Nerve 1998;21:943–5.

135. Vigliani MC, Polo P, Chio A, et al. Patients with amyotrophic lateral sclerosis and cancer do not differ clinically from patients with sporadic amyotrophic lateral sclerosis. J Neurol 2000;247:778–82.
136. Farrell DF, Starr A. Delayed neurological sequelae of electrical injuries. Neurology 1968;18:601–6.
137. Gawel M, Zaiwalla A, Rose FC. Antecedent events in motor neuron disease. J Neurol Neurosurg Psychiatry 1983;46:1041–3.
138. Johansen C, Olsen JH. Mortality from amyotrophic lateral sclerosis, other chronic disorders, and electric shocks among utility workers. Am J Epidemiol 1998;148:362–8.
139. Davanipour Z, Sobel E, Bowman JD, et al. Amyotrophic lateral sclerosis and occupational exposure to electromagnetic fields. Bioelectromagnetics 1997; 18:28–35.
140. Savitz DA, Checkoway H, Loomis DP. Magnetic field exposure and neurodegenerative disease mortality among electric utility workers. Epidemiology 1998;9: 398–404.
141. Savitz DA, Loomis DP, Tse CK. Electrical occupations and neurodegenerative disease: analysis of U.S. mortality data. Arch Environ Health 1998;53:71–4.
142. Noonan CW, Reif JS, Yost M, et al. Occupational exposure to magnetic fields in case-referent studies of neurodegenerative diseases. Scand J Work Environ Health 2002;28:42–8.
143. Håkansson N, Gustavsson P, Johansen C, et al. Neurodegenerative diseases in welders and other workers exposed to high levels of magnetic fields. Epidemiology 2003;14:420–6.
144. Feychting M, Jonsson F, Pedersen NL, et al. Occupational magnetic field exposure and neurodegenerative disease. Epidemiology 2003;14:413–9.
145. Schmidt S, Kwee LC, Allen KD, et al. Association of ALS with head injury, cigarette smoking and APOE genotypes. J Neurol Sci 2010;291:22–9.
146. Savettieri G, Salemi G, Arcara A, et al. A case-control study of amyotrophic lateral sclerosis. Neuroepidemiology 1991;10:242–5.
147. Longstreth WT, McGuire V, Koepsell TD, et al. Risk of amyotrophic lateral sclerosis and history of physical activity: a population-based case-control study. Arch Neurol 1998;55:201–6.
148. Beretta S, Carri MT, Beghi E, et al. The sinister side of Italian soccer. Lancet Neurol 2003;2:656–7.
149. Piazza O, Sirén AL, Ehrenreich H. Soccer, neurotrauma and amyotrophic lateral sclerosis: is there a connection? Curr Med Res Opin 2004;20:505–8.
150. Beghi E, Logroscino G, Chio A, et al. Amyotrophic lateral sclerosis, physical exercise, trauma and sports: results of a population-based pilot case-control study. Amyotroph Lateral Scler 2010;11:289–92.
151. McKee AC, Gavett BE, Stern RA, et al. TDP-43 proteinopathy and motor neuron disease in chronic traumatic encephalopathy. J Neuropathol Exp Neurol 2010; 69:918–29.
152. Turner MR, Abisgold J, Yeates DG, et al. Head and other physical trauma requiring hospitalisation is not a significant risk factor in the development of ALS. J Neurol Sci 2010;288:45–8.
153. Nelson LM, Matkin C, Longstreth WT, et al. Population-based case-control study of amyotrophic lateral sclerosis in western Washington State. II. Diet. Am J Epidemiol 2000;151:164–73.
154. Tylleskär T, Banea M, Bikangi N, et al. Cassava cyanogens and konzo, an upper motoneuron disease found in Africa. Lancet 1992;339(8787):208–11.

155. Caparros-Lefevre D, Elbaz A. Possible relation of atypical parkinsonism in the French West Indies with consumption of tropical plants: a case-control study. Lancet 1999;354:281–6.

156. Morozova N, Weisskopf MG, McCullough ML. Diet and amyotrophic lateral sclerosis. Epidemiology 2008;19:324–37.

157. Mitchell JD. Amyotrophic lateral sclerosis: toxins and environment. Amyotroph Lateral Scler Other Motor Neuron Disord 2000;1:235–50.

158. Kurland LT, Mulder DW. Epidemiologic investigations of amyotrophic lateral sclerosis. 1. Preliminary report on geographic distribution, with special reference to the Mariana Islands, including clinical and pathological observations. Neurology 1954;4:355–78, 438–48.

159. Yoshida S, Uebayashi Y, Kihira T, et al. Epidemiology of motor neuron disease in the Kii Peninsula of Japan, 1989-1993: active or disappearing focus? J Neurol Sci 1998;155:146–55.

160. Anderson FH, Richardson EP, Okazaki H, et al. Neurofibrillary degeneration on Guam: frequency in Chamorros and non Chamorros with no known neurological disease. Brain 1979;102:65–77.

161. Armon C. Environmental risk factors for amyotrophic lateral sclerosis. Neuroepidemiology 2001;20:2–6.

162. Spencer PS, Nunn PB, Hugon J, et al. Motor neuron disease on Guam: possible role of a food neurotoxin. Lancet 1986;1:965.

163. Spencer PS, Nunn PB, Hugon J, et al. Guam amyotrophic lateral sclerosis-parkinsonism-dementia linked to a plant excitant neurotoxin. Science 1987;237:517–22.

164. Zhang ZX, Anderson DW, Mantel N, et al. Motor neuron disease on Guam: geographic and familial occurrence, 1956-85. Acta Neurol Scand 1996;94:51–9.

165. Plato CC, Galasko D, Garruto RM, et al. ALS and PDC of Guam: forty-year follow up. Neurology 2002;58:765–73.

166. Plato CC, Garruto RM, Galasko D, et al. Amyotrophic lateral sclerosis and parkinsonism-dementia complex of Guam: changing incidence rates during the past 60 years. Am J Epidemiol 2003;157:149–57.

167. Whiting MG. Toxicity of cycads. Econ Bot 1963;17:271–302.

168. Duncan MW, Steele JC, Kopin IJ, et al. 2-Amino-3-(methylamino)-propanoic acid (BMAA) in cycad flour: an unlikely cause of amyotrophic lateral sclerosis and parkinsonia-dementia complex of Guam. Neurology 1990;40:767–72.

169. Khabazian I, Bains JS, Williams DE, et al. Isolation of various forms of sterol b-D-glucoside from the seed of *Cycas circinalis*: neurotoxicity and implications for ALS-parkinsonism dementia complex. J Neurochem 2002;82:516–28.

170. Cox PA, Sacks OW. Cycad neurotoxins, consumption of flying foxes, and ALS-PDC disease in Guam. Neurology 2002;58:956–9.

171. Banack SA, Cox PA. Biomagnification of cycad neurotoxins in flying foxes: implications for ALS-PDC in Guam. Neurology 2003;61:387–9.

172. Cox PA, Banack SA, Murch SJ. Biomagnification of cyanobacterial neurotoxins and neurodegenerative disease among the Chamorro people of Guam. Proc Natl Acad Sci U S A 2003;100:13380–3.

173. Murch SJ, Cox PA, Banack SA. A mechanism for slow release of biomagnified cyanobacterial neurotoxins and neurodegenerative disease in Guam. Proc Natl Acad Sci U S A 2004;101:12228–31.

174. Bharucha NE, Schoenberg BS, Raven RH, et al. Geographic distribution of motor neuron disease and correlation with possible etiologic factors. Neurology 1983;33:911–5.

175. Bracco L, Antuono P, Amaducci L. Study of epidemiological and etiological factors of amyotrophic lateral sclerosis in the province of Florence, Italy. Acta Neurol Scand 1979;60:112–24.
176. Minkler M, Fuller-Thomson E, Guralnik JM. Gradient of disability across the socioeconomic spectrum in the United States. N Engl J Med 2006;355:695–703.

Index

Note: Page numbers of article titles are in **boldface** type.

A

Abuse
   drugs of, seizures due to, 541
   methamphetamine, neurologic manifestations of, **641–655.** See also *Methamphetamine, chronic abuse of, neurologic manifestations of.*
Acetylcholine, 550–551
ALS. See *Amyotrophic lateral sclerosis (ALS).*
Aluminum, exposure to, ALS related to, 692
Amine(s), central biogenic, acute excited mental status due to, 546–547
gamma-Aminobutyric acid (GABA), acute depressed mental status due to, 543–544
Amoxapine, 567–568
   overdose-induced seizures due to, 572
Amphetamine(s), acute excited mental status due to, 547
Amyotrophic lateral sclerosis (ALS)
   case studies of, 691
   described, 689–691
   diagnosis of, 690
   educational status and, 701–702
   environmental effects on, **689–711**
      aluminum, 692
      chemicals, 693–695
      cigarette smoking, 695
      diet, 699–700
      electrical shock, 698
      electromagnetic fields, 698
      Gulf War service, 695–696
      heavy metals, 691–693
      infections, 697
      lead, 691–692
      manganese, 693
      mercury, 692
      neoplasms, 697–698
      selenium, 692–693
      solvents, 694–695
      toxins, 693–695
      trace elements, 691–693
   incidence of, 689–690
   physical factors and, 698–699
   prevalence of, 689–690
   socioeconomic status and, 701–702
   Western Pacific, 700–701

Neurol Clin 29 (2011) 713–722
doi:10.1016/S0733-8619(11)00067-3
0733-8619/11/$ – see front matter © 2011 Elsevier Inc. All rights reserved.

neurologic.theclinics.com

Moving?

Make sure your subscription moves with you!

To notify us of your new address, find your **Clinics Account Number** (located on your mailing label above your name), and contact customer service at:

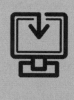

Email: journalscustomerservice-usa@elsevier.com

800-654-2452 (subscribers in the U.S. & Canada)
314-447-8871 (subscribers outside of the U.S. & Canada)

Fax number: 314-447-8029

Elsevier Health Sciences Division
Subscription Customer Service
3251 Riverport Lane
Maryland Heights, MO 63043

*To ensure uninterrupted delivery of your subscription, please notify us at least 4 weeks in advance of move.

Printed and bound by CPI Group (UK) Ltd, Croydon, CR0 4YY

14/10/2024

01773693-0002